POWER
HEALING

POWER HEALING

HEALING

*The Four Keys to
Energizing Your Body,
Mind, and Spirit*

DR. ZHI GANG SHA

HarperSanFrancisco
A Division of HarperCollinsPublishers

HarperCollins books may be purchased for educational, business, or sales promotional use. For information please write: Special Markets Department, HarperCollins Publishers Inc., 10 East 53rd Street, New York, NY 10022.

HarperCollins Web site: http://www.harpercollins.com
HarperCollins®, ☛®, and HarperSanFrancisco™ are trademarks of
HarperCollins Publishers Inc.

FIRST EDITION
Designed by Joseph Rutt

Library of Congress Cataloging-in-Publication Data

Sha, Zhi Gang.
Power healing: the four keys to energizing your body, mind, and spirit /
Zhi Gang Sha.— 1 st ed.
p. cm.
ISBN 0–06–251779–1 (cloth : alk. paper)
1. Qi gong.   2. Medicine, Chinese.   3. Mental healing.   I. Title.
RA781.8 .S477 2001
613.7'1--dc21   2001039757

02 03 04 05 06 ❖/RRD 10 9 8 7 6 5 4 3 2 1

This book is dedicated to all
who want to boost energy for their body, mind, and spirit,
strengthen their immune systems, prevent illness,
improve the quality of their lives, prolong their lives,
relieve pain, including chronic pain,
and recover from illness, including chronic and
life-threatening conditions.

May you find the "Healer Within You"
to self-heal and to heal others,
physically, mentally, emotionally, and spiritually.

CONTENTS

Foreword

In the West, in spite of our tremendous progress we are experiencing a medical crisis. Even the most conservative doctors agree that people have become too dependent on their doctors and medications to stay healthy. No matter how competent or big our medical system becomes, it cannot completely heal us or keep us healthy. Gradually we have given away our power to heal ourselves. Ideally, healing should be our job. Doctors and remedies can help, but we should be doing more of the work.

It is hard to take back our power to self-heal when we are faced in all directions with the latest breakthrough diet or health program. Even the experts often directly contradict each other. There are so many choices that it is hard to know what to do. Having choices is a great gift, but it also brings additional stress. And the more we depend on remedies outside ourselves to solve the problem, the greater our stress becomes. This burden, however, is significantly lessened when we learn the secrets of how to heal ourselves.

Taking back the responsibility to heal ourselves is the answer to our health-care crisis. As we learn to awaken within ourselves our natural self-healing ability, we no longer feel confused about which health program is right for us. We gain confidence in our ability to heal ourselves and in finding and working with the assistance of the programs that are available.

Doctors continually find that what works for one patient doesn't work for another. It is often a mystery why one program works for many but not all. The answer to this question lies in understanding how the body heals itself, which the body is actually perfectly designed to do. That is why some people stay healthy. When we get sick, a part of our natural self-healing response is blocked or suppressed in some manner. If we first learn to awaken our natural self-healing response when we become sick, modern medicine and other alternative healing methods have a better chance of helping us return to health.

Modern medicine has clearly made many miraculous strides and advances. Yet each great step or new advance can take us only so far; we eventually reach our limit and begin searching anew for answers. Often that search sends us back to earlier theories. This is the nature of progress. Only after we have stepped ahead can we reach back into our past, reassess what we left behind, and use it to enrich our new discoveries. We are now fortunate to be living at a time when the ancient knowledge and wisdom of most cultures is available at our fingertips. This ancient knowledge contains many jewels of wisdom that, with a little adjusting here and there, can be immensely helpful to reawaken our self-healing ability.

Already doctors in the West have come to recognize the amazing benefits of five-thousand-year-old traditional Chinese medicine. Most recognized is the value of Chinese acupuncture. Volumes of research have now been done to validate its effectiveness in treating a long list of sicknesses and diseases. What is not known so well are the secrets of self-healing.

Many of these secrets were even withheld from the Chinese public. In ancient days, most ordinary people in China were only knowledgeable about the beginning techniques. As a result, they depended more on acupuncture and herbs to treat sickness and stay healthy. Yet there were always a select few who were more advanced in their consciousness and knowledge. These older souls, often called masters, were capable of doing advanced self-healing techniques and were not dependent on doctors, herbs, or acupuncture. Practicing secret self-healing techniques, they lived to be well beyond a hundred years old without getting sick. Many of these ancient secrets are being brought to the public's attention for the first time in Dr. Zhi Gang Sha's *Power Healing: The Four Keys to Energizing Your Body, Mind, and Spirit.*

Great masters and teachers of all traditions have always spoken of a time when the secrets would come forth, a time when humankind would be able to comprehend the higher truths about life so that everyone could live together in health, justice, and harmony. That time is now here. The shift has taken place.

Over the past thirty years while teaching and developing the ideas of *Men Are from Mars, Women Are from Venus*, I also continued to practice and teach a variety of self-healing techniques that I learned from various traditions and teachings. In my own personal search to find "enlightenment" and literally heal the blindness in my left eye, I have traveled around the world over twenty times.

I have studied with great masters and healers of nearly all the great traditions, including the Christian, Jewish, Muslim, Sufi, Hindu, Buddhist, Mayan, Incan, and Chinese traditions. In my own way, I have sifted through these many approaches and used what worked for me. The result was clearly a blessed life with much love and success, and, yes, my blindness was healed. Because of my years of disciplined practice, I was given access to many of the most advanced techniques, which I, in kind, kept secret.

About three years ago I began to notice that the self-healing results people were getting had become much more profound than in years before. I discovered that people progressed more quickly in these different practices when they skipped the beginning techniques and went straight to the advanced techniques.

A wonderful shift had taken place. Beginners' techniques were no longer needed and the advanced techniques worked right away for everyone. Ironically, when the student is ready, the advanced techniques are much more simple than beginning ones. People in my healing workshops were having experiences that had taken me twenty-five years of devoted practice to attain.

I discovered that people today only need access to the secret advanced techniques, and they can suddenly experience the benefits that in the past only the masters have enjoyed. In times past, these advanced techniques were kept secret only because they would not work for the ordinary person, but that is not the case anymore.

Dr. Sha has spent his life studying and mastering the different healing modalities of traditional Chinese medicine. He is himself a pathway between the West and the East. He is a Western medical doctor as well as a traditional Chinese medicine expert, including herbalist, acupuncturist, and qigong master. He was featured in the spring 2000 PBS documentary entitled "Qigong: Ancient Chinese Healing for the 21st Century." He is a self-healing pioneer who has trained thousands of people to heal themselves of chronic conditions. His vibrant, powerful, revolutionary techniques bring new understanding to the relationship between illness and health.

He also has discovered that at this time in history the ancient self-healing secrets reserved only for the masters can now be taught effectively to everyone. Dr. Sha makes available secret techniques and insights that were only available in the past to a select few. He shares in simple terms the insights and tools that took him more than thirty years of hard work and discipline to attain. He gives you access to information and techniques that would otherwise be unattainable.

I have personally benefited from many of Dr. Sha's power-healing secrets. In one session, with his assistance in a workshop, I released the chronic pain I had experienced in both my feet. At a later workshop, during allergy season, with his assistance I was able to radically minimize my allergy reactions. Then, after two weeks they disappeared completely. I had been plagued by allergies for my entire life. In his workshops, I also witnessed a wide range of miraculous results, from healing chronic pain, depression, and arthritis to accelerating the recovery time for cancer.

The time has come to awaken your hidden potential for self-healing. If you are suffering from chronic pain or other unhealthy conditions, Dr. Sha's *Power Healing* will help you begin to heal yourself. These simple and practical techniques can be used by young and old, laypeople and professionals. Use them to self-heal physical, mental, emotional, and spiritual conditions. Test out these techniques for yourself and find what works for you. Use these simple and practical self-healing tools to restore your health and enjoy your God-given birthright.

Dr. John Gray

INTRODUCTION

Do you, your family members, or friends suffer from physical, emotional, mental, or spiritual health problems? Do any of you suffer from chronic pain or illness, or even from life-threatening conditions such as cancer? Even if you are healthy, would you like to have more energy and stamina? Would you like to strengthen your immune system?

If you have any of these health concerns, how do you deal with them? Have you heard about self-healing? Self-healing means that you help to restore your own health. Do you know about self-healing through energy work, spiritual healing, or other methods?

Do you realize that your body has its own capacity to self-heal? Do you realize that if you activate your own self-healing capabilities, you will recover much faster? Do you realize that all other kinds of healing are not complete without self-healing?

I offer you the essence of self-healing, from five thousand years of Chinese culture, including energy healing and spiritual healing practices. The four keys to power healing that I present to you in this book are body power (special standing, sitting, and hand positions), sound power (special healing sounds and mantras), mind power (guided imagery and creative visualizations), and soul power (soul communication and soul healing). Parts of these techniques have been practiced successfully by millions of people in China to self-heal and heal others throughout its five-thousand-year history. They have never been revealed in their entirety to the public before. They are secrets to people in the West. They are secrets even to the Chinese people, because these secrets have been hidden and practiced only by the masters. A master may pass the deep understanding and insights of these techniques to only one or two chosen disciples in his or her lifetime.

To master the knowledge and deep insights of the four keys to power healing, I have devoted almost forty years to serious study of many Chinese cultural arts and sciences, including tai chi, qigong, feng shui, Buddhism, Taoism, and Confucianism. I am a doctor of traditional Chinese medicine and also an M.D. in Western medicine.

People in all parts of the world have practiced power-healing techniques, such as creative visualizations, mantras, and body movements, without realizing the power of combining all of them. One morning in April 1995, I was practicing some self-healing exercises using power-healing techniques. Suddenly, in a single moment, I understood that the four keys to power healing could be applied and practiced together. Applying a single technique for healing is powerful, but applying all four together is much more powerful. This is the first time that all four keys to power healing have been combined and disclosed.

This is the wisdom of ancient China, preserved, practiced, and presented to the whole world. Now, at the beginning of the twenty-first century, it is the right time for me to share these secrets with you. At the dawn of this new millennium, my masters have sent me to the West with the authority to spread this knowledge to the public, to serve people in the entire world. The purpose of this book is to provide you with powerful self-healing and healing tools for body, mind, and soul.

Many of you seek relief from physical pain and emotional imbalance. You may be mentally confused or lack spiritual direction. You may be suffering. You try to get well, seeking out doctors, healers, and a variety of other healing specialists. Power healing is the approach you need for self-healing. Power healing vitalizes self-healing, just as eating food, drinking water, and breathing air vitalize life itself. In my practice and workshops, I have taught many people how to improve their health, habits, and lives by incorporating these simple, quick, effective, and powerful self-healing methods into their daily lives.

Power healing can also be used to assist doctors in helping their patients and in conjunction with any and all conventional medical practices and complementary and alternative health methods. Combine the four keys to power healing with advice and help from your doctor or healer. I have no conflict with medical professionals. I am simply advocating self-healing and self-responsibility.

Power-healing techniques can assist all doctors and healers. Power healing is compatible with all kinds of medicine and healing methods, including Western medicine, traditional Chinese medicine, complementary medicine, alternative medicine, Ayurvedic medicine, and native and indigenous medicine.

Power healing will help you discover and understand your relationship with your own health. You will come to know the "healer within you."

Many of you have been searching for self-healing knowledge and techniques, searching for well-being. You are searching for ways to be healthier and happier. You want more satisfaction in your lives. You may want spiritual enlightenment as well. As I have studied, learned, and taught, I have grown from a student to become a master. At the same time, I have always remained a student and continue to learn more. I fully understand now that it is not necessary for anyone to take twenty or thirty years to learn the four keys to power healing. I present to you the essence of power healing, an essence that is simple, practical, powerful, and profound. Anyone can learn power-healing techniques and receive their benefits to heal body, mind, and soul right away.

Five thousand years ago, traditional Chinese medicine concluded that every sickness is caused by an imbalance of *chi*. *Chi* (pronounced "chee") means "vital energy" and "life force." Power healing works because its techniques stimulate cellular vibration and promote *chi* flow at the cellular level. Each power-healing technique alone can stimulate cellular vibration but, used together, the four keys to power healing accelerate cellular vibration. This acceleration brings healing results much faster, because the promotion of *chi* flow helps to remove energy blockages, which strengthens your immune system, restores your health, improves the quality of your life, and prolongs your life.

Best of all, power healing is simple. In my forty-year study journey, I have come to understand that the most powerful healing methods are the simplest methods. If you have an energy blockage in your body, the power-healing techniques will help you remove the blockage and restore your well-being. Although simple and practical, power healing is powerful. It can bring healing results quickly, even immediately. As you read this book, you will find many examples of the powerful effect of using the four keys to power healing together. I will also give you clear explanations of why these techniques work.

With so much suffering and limited medical resources, more and more of you are seeking to learn and practice self-healing to augment the services you get from medical professionals and alternative health practitioners. Your need for medical services is great. Your interest in alternative services and self-healing is growing. In response to this growing interest, PBS, the Public Broadcasting System in the United States, presented a one-hour documentary entitled "Qigong: Ancient Chinese Healing for the 21st Century" in the spring of 2000. The documentary, produced by Francesco Garripoli, president of the Qigong Institute, featured my teacher, Master and Dr. Zhi Chen Guo, and me in China. It is my sincere wish that this book will satisfy the thirst for the knowledge behind the remarkable self-healing techniques shown in that film.

My mission is to serve all of you by empowering you with the tools to heal yourselves and others on the physical, mental, emotional, and spiritual levels and to help you increase your spiritual awareness and achieve soul enlightenment. Open this book to find the self-healing knowledge, methods, and techniques that you need for health. Apply the methods and use the techniques by following the clear and simple instructions in this book. Feel the healing blessings that will come to you. Develop great self-healing power by practicing the four keys to power healing together. Try it. Heal yourself. These power-healing techniques are waiting to serve you.

It is my great honor to bring the message of the four keys to power healing to the world. Enjoy a healthy body, intelligent mind, and enlightened soul by practicing power healing in your daily life.

1

HELP YOURSELF

Despite continual advances in medical technology and know-how, incidences of illness and pain in this country are on the rise. Hypertension is rampant. The number of deaths from heart disease and stroke is rising instead of falling. Every other person you meet seems to be suffering from chronic pain caused by arthritis or bursitis or some other "-itis," and cancer is striking way too close to home. If that isn't bad enough, each allergy and flu season seems worse than the last.

So why do we get sick or fall victim to pain? Western medicine believes that sickness is caused by invasive elements (including bacteria, viruses, and parasites), inherited conditions, or injury. Pain and incurable disease are often chalked up to aging or chance. But that doesn't explain why we are vulnerable in some cases, but not in others. Nor does it explain why some of us succumb to whatever comes near us, while others never seem to get sick at all.

I have a different theory, one that has led to vanquishing everything from colds and allergies to, for some, seemingly incurable diseases and to alleviating even the most chronic pain. The explanation behind why our bodies—and even our mental and emotional health—fall into disrepair is quite simple. Indeed, it can be summed up in a single word: energy.

You can feel your body's field of energy simply by holding your palms as close together as you can without letting them actually touch. Feel the heat? You've just felt the energy that radiates from the cellular vibrations of your skin, tendons, muscles, and blood vessels. In short, you've just felt what the Chinese call *chi* (pronounced "chee")—your vital energy or life force. In a tightly controlled experiment conducted in 1992 at Beijing's China National Radio and Television Research Laboratory, twenty doctors and scientists saw an individual's emission of energy—of *chi*—actually register on the ultrasensitive laboratory equipment.

Healthy energy in the body—*chi*—stems from the healthy vibration of cells in every single part of you. When that vibration is in perfect order, your body has a good flow of energy. If that energy becomes blocked, imbalanced, or diverted, pain or illness results.

It doesn't matter whether we get sick on a physical, emotional, or spiritual level. All sickness begins at the cellular level. Cells are constantly vibrating, contracting and expanding. In the process of contracting and expanding, matter transforms to energy and energy back to matter. When cells contract, it's as if the cells are breathing out. Matter is released and transforms to energy. Conversely, when cells expand, it's as though cells are breathing in. Energy is taken from outside the cells and transforms to matter inside the cells.

So how does this relate to energy problems and getting sick or being in pain?

If cells contract too much or don't expand enough, then too much energy is released in the spaces around the cells. This accumulated excess energy around the cells will not be in balance with the matter inside the cells. This imbalance causes problems like inflammation, pain, and even cancer.

On the other hand, when cells expand too much, they take too much energy from around the cells and convert that energy to matter inside the cells. So you wind up with too much matter inside the cells and insufficient energy outside the cells. This imbalance causes problems like chronic fatigue and other degenerative diseases such as Alzheimer's.

So how does this apply to you? What if I told you that you could access a system that would:

- Develop energy throughout your body—throughout your main internal organs as well as your main energy centers
- Balance energy in your body, mind, and soul
- Release chronic pain
- Improve the functioning of your immune system
- Help heal illness
- Improve stamina and overall health
- Improve the quality of your life

You can. Even better, you don't have to depend on anyone but yourself to gain these benefits.

Energy in your body can be moved, and you can do it. Using the four keys to power healing presented in this book, you can stimulate cellular vibration, remove blockages, and direct energy flow in a healthy pattern.

The fact is that we all have the power to heal ourselves. I can do it. You can do it. And you can do it better. You are the healer.

The concepts, theories, methods, and techniques introduced in this book are simple, practical, powerful, and profound. These self-healing tools can help you correct unhealthy conditions at the physical, emotional, and spiritual levels, thereby enabling you to become more responsible for your own health. If you're already under the care of a doctor or psychologist or receiving any other type of healing service, the techniques you're about to learn will support and complement your other treatments and restore your physical, emotional, and/or mental health even faster.

If you're fortunate enough to have good health, you'll learn how to improve your immune system and quality of life. You'll learn how to prolong that life. You can even learn how to change your environment to improve your health and energy. People pay thousands of dollars to bring in feng shui masters to move their furniture in order to create better energy flow in their homes or offices. But just by sitting in a room, you'll be able to tell whether you feel serene and at ease or uptight and edgy. It's all about paying attention to what's going on around you and inside of you, and then taking the appropriate steps to improve the energy flow.

In the past, we've been content to let experts dictate how to make us well or pain free, and they've done that with varying degrees of success. Ultimately, however, you are the best arbiter of what's going on with your body, and you are the one best suited to fix it. So why sit in the passenger seat of your own physical, mental, and emotional health? Once you've learned how, you can move over and drive yourself.

2

EAST MEETS WEST

The West has a lot to learn from the East. Only recently, for example, has Western medicine recognized stress and tension as causative factors for physical—as well as emotional and mental—illnesses. Traditional Chinese medicine, on the other hand, has always believed that sickness is caused by three factors: natural external factors, internal factors, and accidental factors.

Natural external factors such as wind, cold, summer heat, dampness, dryness, and fire are considered the first cause of sickness. Everybody knows that when it's cold, people easily catch cold, get sore throats, headaches, runny noses, bronchitis, and pneumonia. When the weather is dry, people have more nosebleeds and dry, chapped skin. In very hot weather, the heart beats faster. You might have difficulty breathing or suffer dizziness. Heart trouble may flare up. Dampness and fog in cities such as San Francisco and London cause people to have arthritis and joint pain.

The *internal factors* that cause ill health are mainly emotional conditions, such as anger, overexcitement, sadness, worry, grief, and fear. You can see the connection for yourself the next time you get very angry. I promise you, though you may reach for a plate to throw at someone, you won't be thinking about eating off of it, because you'll have no desire to eat at all. That's because emotional anger stimulates the liver cells, causing the cells to vibrate too much. Then, lots of energy radiates out of the liver. That energy puts pressure on the stomach, causing a feeling of fullness. That's why a person with great anger has no appetite and does not want to eat. After great anger, some people even suffer a stroke. Why does this happen? The anger strongly vibrates the liver cells, causing too much energy to radiate out from the liver and flow up to the head. The sudden accumulation of this energy can cause high blood pressure that can result in a stroke.

Try to think about your own experience or the experiences of family members and friends when they have experienced great anger. Their face grows red, and their head feels like it's about to burst. That makes sense, since so much energy has accumulated in the head.

Last among traditional Chinese medicine's explanations for sickness are *accidental factors* such as accidents, snakebites, or traumatic injuries. Even here, however, these causative agents are looked at in conjunction with the person as a whole.

This radically different way of looking at illness and pain affects both diagnosis and treatment decisions.

Western medical diagnosis is based on physiological, pathological, and anatomical evaluation and depends upon the complaints of the patient, general observation, family history, physical examination and tests, and diagnostic tools such as X rays, sonograms, and CAT scans. Once the problem has been identified, Western medical treatment attempts to change the matter (not the energy) of the human body by means of instruments, such as in laser treatments and surgery, and/or through biochemical matter, including drugs, intravenous solutions, and ointments.

Diagnosis by traditional Chinese medicine depends upon the signs and symptoms collected by observation, inquiry, listening, smelling, and pulse reading. In keeping with its theoretical foundation of conceiving of the organism as a whole, all signs and symptoms (physical, mental, emotional, and spiritual) are analyzed to find the root, nature, and location of disease. Treatment then adjusts and restores the body's functions by using natural means, such as herbs and acupuncture, to transform matter to energy and vice versa. "In contradistinction to most Western medicine in which we classify and diagnose disease and not the person, Chinese medicine, like most psychotherapies, is concerned with an individual's unique physical and emotional state," writes Leon Hammer, M.D., in his book *Dragon Rises, Red Bird Flies*. "Treating . . . symptoms and signs without reading in them the story of the person is a denial of the role which the patient plays in his or her own disharmony."[1]

In the Eastern scheme, ill health results from disharmony or imbalance in the body's energy system. Finding the source of that imbalance is the key to treatment. Hammer goes on to explain:

The underlying "cause" as expressed by character and behavior patterns, and not by the "symptom," is the focus. The "cause," as we use the term, is not an outside invading force, a virus or bacterium; rather, it is intrinsic to the individual and the lifestyle he or she generates.

Chinese medicine regards a symptom as a signal of unattended, underlying issues and not as a disagreeable phenomenon to be eliminated. Symptoms are opportunities to examine one's life, to reconsider one's values and habits, to re-evaluate one's personality and relationships, to expand awareness, and to change. . . . The goal of Chinese medicine is prevention of illness through the knowledge of natural law, which includes altering oneself so as to live in greater harmony with that law.[2]

Although some of this may sound complicated, the bottom line is simply this. Imagine your body having the potential to resist disease and repel infection no matter what it's exposed to! Imagine a treatment that works to shore up your body's defenses instead of triggering its resistance to the latest drug you're being given. Now close your eyes and imagine having the ability to tap into this treatment at will, without being dependent on anything or anybody to provide it.

You can do more than dream about it. You can live it, just as Paul does.

In 1998, Paul's life was shattered when he was abruptly fired after moving his family halfway across the country in order to take a new job as a business development manager for a software company. An avid skier, martial arts fanatic, basketball jock, and national chess champion who had always excelled at what he undertook, Paul felt like a failure. Unused to a lack of success of any kind, his self-esteem plummeted. So did his health. First came the colds, flus, and other associated illnesses. Then the thirty-four-year-old came down with a viral infection that led to a massive asthma attack that shut down his lungs and nearly took his life.

The fierce attack scared him, especially since it seemed to come out of the blue. In hindsight, he had ignored the subtle warning signs his body provided, like his allergies becoming more pronounced. But the allergies never seemed to affect his breathing, and so this stress-induced escalation really blindsided him.

When Paul was finally released from the hospital, his doctor said he was lucky to be alive. He didn't need to be told. During the next three years, Paul attempted to control his condition.

Though conventional medicine has concluded that asthma is not curable, he refused to accept that conclusion.

Initially, he worked closely with a pulmonalogist who prescribed six medications. However, the oral steroids often made him nauseous, and the lack of progress was downright frustrating. Despite all his efforts, he seemed to repeat the same cycle, taking ill every three or four months. Flu season was the scariest time of all, with bad attacks hitting hard every winter.

As the months turned into years, Paul's hope began to dim, and he grew increasingly depressed. Ironically, that proved a blessing. A disciplined person who had trained himself to focus his attention like a laser on his illness, he began to notice that when his negative thoughts increased, his health worsened. Noticing the pattern, however, wasn't enough to alter it. As his health deteriorated, he became even more depressed, which further compromised his health. Unable to see a way out of this downward spiral, he watched his entire lifestyle disintegrate before his eyes.

Then, in October 2000, he met me and began to study my self-healing techniques. The more he practiced them, the more his lungs cleared and his energy returned. Even his digestion improved, which surprised him. He had not known how closely connected digestion is to the lungs.

"I realized that I can help my body," Paul says. "The results were immediate, yet the techniques seemed so simple that I wanted to practice them even more. It was wonderful to experience more energy and enthusiasm as a result. I realized that the most challenging problems usually have the simplest solution, but I had no idea that the key to achieving mental and physical health was so simple and elegant."

Paul had made great strides toward helping himself. Still, a month after he'd started to learn how to self-heal, he fell ill again with a bad virus. Just as he seemed to come out of it with only minor difficulties, an asthma attack suddenly struck in the middle of the night. Though he immediately took the necessary fast-acting medication, the condition grew worse. Finally, his wife took him to the hospital. The emergency room was packed, with a wait that could last hours. Paul started to sweat. He knew all too well that once his condition deteriorated beyond a certain point, the situation could become critical within a few minutes.

Instead of panicking, however, he decided to try what he'd learned with me. First he asked his body to relax and for his lungs to help themselves to clear away the inflammation. Then he started to chant "Ar Mi Tuo Fuo" almost silently, his wife accompanying him in a low voice. (I will explain this great mantra in Chapter 8.) The emergency room grew more hectic by the minute with incoming patients. But within about ten minutes his lungs began to discharge phlegm, which he was able to cough out. The discharge continued for an hour. When he was finally admitted to see the doctor an hour and a half later, he needed no intervention. Never before had his lungs reversed themselves once an attack had started. But this time, "my lungs solved the problem themselves!" he says. "Though prior asthmatic emergencies had even required my being resuscitated after technically dying, I no longer needed treatment of any kind and was able to walk right out of the hospital."

"The message I wish to convey from this story is one of hope," he adds. "It feels wonderful to be confident that I am in control of my health and well-being."

The Chinese have long known that people with all kinds of sicknesses can learn to activate the body's healing power. The result? A reduction in hospitalization time and cost, less need for medications, and greater healing in diseases ranging from hypertension to cancer.

Over the centuries, different aspects of the knowledge I'm

about to share with you have been kept secret—by masters, who could pass their deep understanding and insights to only one or two chosen disciples in their lifetime, by the upper class, and by warriors who used it to give themselves the advantage on the battlefield. This is the first time they've been combined into a single powerful healing system.

"You never really know how you are going to take the news that you are terminally ill, not treatable, and that you are going to die," says Jerry, a fifty-eight-year-old engineer and former manager of a telecommunications company who was diagnosed four and a half years ago with colon cancer that had metastasized to his lung and liver. Sentenced to thirteen months of chemotherapy, he was told that he should prepare to die anyway.

"Despite the news, I was not horrified," he says. "My engineering training had taught me to be highly analytical and very skeptical and that everything needed proof. I basically did not accept what my doctor was telling me. At an early age I began investigating miracles, metaphysics, and spirituality, so I knew exceptions existed to everything. Many people say they meditate and don't, but I really do. In fact, I have been meditating twice a day for twenty to thirty minutes each day since 1972. Over thirty years of meditation and studying ancient literature and metaphysical Bible teachings are probably the reason I am alive today.

"Still, my doctor's news that April 17, 1997, was about as bad as it gets. A strong knowing came over me from my studies that nothing happens by accident and that whatever happens happens for a reason. 'You'll be fine,' I heard a loud, resounding, reassuring voice announce, negating what my doctor was telling me. I needed all my scientific, analytical, and management skills to simply maneuver my way through the medical system maze. Along the way, I decided to explore alternative treatments to accompany the chemotherapy. That's when I discovered self-healing from Dr. Sha.

"What a difference! First, I could see results from these simple, practical techniques, results that stemmed from my actions. As my health improved and my dependency on my doctors lessened, I felt increasingly empowered and self-reliant. The self-healing techniques have helped my wife and me to relieve our sore throats. My energy has increased. And most important, when I went back to my doctor for my CEA count [tumor marker count], which is determined by a blood test and then a series of routine follow-up tests, for the first time in five years my counts were normal. What a relief! A 77 percent reduction!

"I was totally amazed, but not as amazed as my doctor seemed to be. Two months ago I had a CAT scan that showed no sign of tumors in my lungs, liver, or colon. Recently my CEA level began to go up again, so it's time to get busy again. But I have every confidence.

"Five years ago, my doctor told me that I could expect to die soon. But I'm still alive, feeling healthy, and enjoying my retirement. I hike, I go to movies, I watch comedies, I meditate, and I continue to explore natural self-healing practices."

3

GO WITH THE FLOW

Everyone has a self-healing system. You've seen that for yourself many times in your own body. Think about the last time you cut yourself or twisted a knee or an ankle. You may have elevated the wound, applied ice, or rested your injury. But basically your cut closed itself up without much conscious help from you, just as the swelling in your afflicted joint diminished and eventually disappeared, along with the pain. If you've broken a bone, you know that the cast is just there to keep the bone securely in place so that it can knit itself back together again.

Even antibiotics, considered by most to be an astonishing, albeit overused, "miracle cure," may merely serve to diminish the number of bacteria, thereby allowing the immune system to carry on with its job and eliminate an infection.

Your body has the unparalleled ability to heal itself if given half a chance. In many cases, however, the body doesn't even have to work that hard. Research conducted by the U.S. Department of Health and Human Services reveals that an astounding 70 percent of all illness is actually avoidable. Instead of engaging in mortal combat with the enemy, most of us can sidestep the battle completely simply by pumping up our immune systems.

Unblocking and moving energy through cellular vibration is the key.

Biology defines the cell as the smallest independently functioning unit of the human body. A cell consists of membrane, nucleus, cytoplasm, DNA, RNA, mitochondria, and other organelles. Every internal organ and tissue in the body consists of cells. Living cells have various functions, such as protection, secretion, immune duties, reproduction, absorption, and elimination.

In addition to performing their various functions, cells vibrate. They expand, contract, spin, wobble, twist, and rock nonstop, sort of like peripatetic teenagers. Some movements are consistent, others random. But any and all of this activity radiates energy.

Although Western medicine does study biochemical changes in cells, it doesn't pay much attention to cell vibration or cell energy with respect to health. Yet in my view, getting—and staying—healthy starts right here. Matter inside the cells and energy outside the cells are constantly transforming, each into the other. When a person is healthy, this transformation between matter and energy remains in relative balance. Any factor that causes an imbalance in this transformation results in illness.

I remind you that when cells expand, they breathe in the energy around them and transform this energy into internal matter. When cells contract, they breathe out, thereby transforming the matter inside them to energy around them.

Remember how you could feel the heat when you held your palms very close together? What you were feeling was the transformation of matter from inside the cells of your palms into energy outside the cells of your palms.

It's like a dance that's happening inside you all the time. Every once in a while, however, elements such as bacteria, viruses, anger, worry, grief, or accidents can throw a kink into this dynamic two-step by creating an imbalance in the transformation between matter inside the cells and energy outside the cells. That's when you get sick. To get well, you must restore that balance. To stay well, you must increase your energy so that it's less vulnerable to those elements that can affect it.

Cells vibrate more strongly when you develop your energy. They also tend to vibrate in balanced patterns that support good health. When cells vibrate strongly, they influence nearby cells to vibrate in the same way. This phenomenon, known as sympathetic vibration, encourages all the cells in your body to vibrate in the same healthy patterns. You can even encourage another person's cells to vibrate in accordance with your healthy patterns if your energy is highly developed.

Overactive cells, however, will create too much energy in one area of your body. When the accumulated energy grows too great to be transmitted to other parts of the body, a blockage occurs.

Imagine a river. The river level rises after a heavy rain. If the volume of water is too great for the channel, the river starts to spill over its banks. Water then pools on the surrounding land and stagnates. Diseases start spreading.

Energy can accumulate in the body in much the same way. When energy doesn't flow properly in the body, conditions for poor health are established. Overvibrating cells may result in acute or chronic pain, inflammation, infection, hemorrhage, heart attack, stroke, cysts, unusual growths, tumors, and hyperactivity of the organs.

Factors such as weather, pollution, and emotions can also cause cells to vibrate too slowly. The result? These undervibrating cells don't radiate enough energy to sustain healthy functioning. Symptoms may include hypofunctioning (underactivity) of the organs, fatigue, reduced immune function, Alzheimer's disease, osteoporosis, edema, and weakness.

Just as cells consist of matter, so do organs. Like cells, organs are also constantly vibrating, expanding and contracting, breathing in energy (transforming energy to matter) and breathing out (transforming matter back to energy).

Yes, it's another dance. But the dancing doesn't stop here, because once the matter from the cell or the organ has transformed back to energy, it radiates back and forth in the cell field (the space around each cell) or the organ field (the space around each organ), colliding and mixing to form new energy. (Picture a rave, with a bunch of young kids body slamming, and you'll get the idea.) New energy is always being produced, energy that will transform back to matter inside the different organs or cells.

So how does all this apply to you? Let's say you get a cold-related sore throat. The bacteria or virus that caused the infection is now stimulating the cells in your throat to make them vibrate more than usual. This means that your overactive throat cells are now radiating more energy than can be absorbed or dissipated by the neighboring tissues and organs. The result is blocked energy in your throat, which manifests itself as the raw throat that's making you miserable. The solution? To rebalance the energy flow in that area, thereby reducing the soreness and inflammation.

Though the diagnoses and treatments used by Western medicine and traditional Chinese medicine appear to be very different, I believe that the essence of all healing practices is to balance the transformation between matter inside the cells and energy outside the cells.

The self-healing techniques in this book work well because they stimulate the vibration of the cells in order to balance the transformation between the matter inside the cells and the energy outside the cells. Since all unhealthy conditions arise from an imbalance in this transformation, restoring your energy balance and flow is what restores your health.

When you think about it, that's all acupuncture does. Now so widely accepted for its preventative and healing abilities that even health insurance companies are covering its costs, this method simply entails sticking needles into somebody's body to stimulate and rebalance the flow of energy. Sound familiar?

Yoga and tai chi constitute other ways to accomplish this same goal. By stretching and moving your body, you disperse energy blockages. But there are other ways to move energy—through hand positions that use simple principles from physics, mantras that stimulate vibration internally, visualization, and more.

That's where I come in.

4

How I Learned the Four Keys to Power Healing

In this life, I started my learning journey at the age of six. I have clear memories of growing up in Xian, Shaanxi Province, China. Xian is an important city in ancient Chinese history. Many emperors made Xian their capital. Xian is well known today because it is near the tomb of Qin Shi Huang, the emperor who first united China. This tomb is one of the great wonders of the world because of the life-sized terra-cotta warriors and horses found buried there.

One morning, my parents took me to the park to play. In a secluded corner among many trees, I watched an old master practicing body motions with his three disciples. The disciples followed each movement as he demonstrated tai chi. He showed his disciples the "Touching Hands" movement. Just a slight touch from the old master's hand would propel a student fifteen feet away. My heart jumped. "Wow!" I thought. "This man is such a powerful master." I stared at him with eyes wide open.

During a break in the routine, I ran to the master and said, "*Ye Ye* ('Grandfather,' used as a sign of respect when greeting any senior gentleman), could you teach me? I would like to learn from you."

He said, "You are such a little boy! You are so young to be interested in learning this."

I said, "Oh yes, *Ye Ye,* I really want to learn."

There must have been a mind or soul connection there because the master instantly became interested in me also. He said, "If you want to learn, I must see your parents."

I was so excited. I turned around, ran to my parents, and pulled them by the hands to see the master. "Oh, I am so excited! Ba Ba, Ma Ma, I want to learn this!"

The master and my parents conferred. My parents then told him, "We give our permission and our support for our son to learn from you."

From that moment on, I started tai chi practice. Each Saturday and Sunday, I was brought to the park to receive training. The master showed me all 108 tai chi positions. For each position, he taught me the health benefits and the self-defense secrets.

At age ten, I met a qigong master. I was as interested in this ancient art as I was in tai chi. I studied very hard and became dedicated to qigong. It has been a lifelong study for me. I learned Shaolin kung fu with knife, sword, and stick. Later, I became a special disciple of Professor Da Jun Liu, a world-renowned I Ching and feng shui master.

I have been a disciple of the Buddhist master Wu Yi, who is one of the most respected Buddhist fathers in the world. Continuing in my study and learning journey, I studied traditional Chinese medicine and Western medicine at Xian Medical University, where I received my M.D. degree.

I then studied with the founder of Zhi Neng medicine, Master and Dr. Zhi Chen Guo. *Zhi Neng* means "intelligence and capabilities of the mind and soul." As you will see, Zhi Neng medicine is a hybrid of ancient Chinese and modern Western healing philosophies and practices. I have learned the most about energy and spiritual healing from Master Guo.

Zhi Neng medical training allowed me to develop the capability to communicate directly with spiritual teachers in the spiritual world. Slowly, I began to receive knowledge directly from these teachers. It took many years of study and practice to gain greater access to this knowledge. This discipline is rigorous, and its benefits may seem mysterious to those unfamiliar with this realm.

At the beginning of my studies, I began to understand *chi*. I experienced it as a warm feeling that flowed through my arms and legs. My whole body would feel warm. When I started my qigong journey at age ten, I learned a mantra that I repeated again and again, for many hours a day. My teacher told me: "Practice the mantra. It is good for gaining power." This became the only idea in my head. My teacher also taught me creative visualization. I would sit and do the exercises as he taught me, but did not really understand why we did the visualizations.

It was only after studying Buddhist and Taoist teaching, Confucian philosophy and Lao Tse's *Tao Te Jing* that I began to understand spiritual principles and laws. My understanding grew as my studies deepened. Although I learned more about the spiritual journey and enlightenment, I did not yet have a clear picture of the four keys to power healing.

When I went to study Western medicine at Xian Medical University, I wanted to understand as much as I could about how Western medicine dealt with sickness, health, and healing. After earning my M.D. degree, I understood that Western medicine has many advantages, for example, the value to the patient of clear diagnosis, readily available emergency care, regular physical checkups, and public-health programs that offer immunizations.

For chronic illness and pain, such as migraines, lower back pain, fatigue, arthritis, and many other health conditions, I found that Western medicine does not provide enough help. I became more interested in traditional Chinese medicine, since it has been practiced by millions of people in China for five thousand years with good results for chronic pain and illness. My study of traditional Chinese medicine included acupuncture, Chinese massage, and the use of Chinese herbs. I also studied energy and spiritual healing methods from other disciplines.

Beginning in 1949, the Chinese government launched a program to combine Western medicine with traditional Chinese medicine. They continued this effort for more than forty years without success. The Eastern and Western systems appear to be completely different. As a student, I wondered, "Is there a theory or a medical system that can combine both Western and traditional Chinese medicine?" My study and learning journey has been a search to find the secrets that could combine these great systems and even go beyond them.

In 1986, the Chinese Ministry of Health sent me to a master's degree program in hospital administration at the University of the Philippines on a World Health Organization scholarship. While I was in school, my father sent me a book titled *Dong Yi Gong*, written by Master and Dr. Zhi Chen Guo, the founder of Zhi Neng medicine. Literally, *Dong* means "using," *Yi* means "thinking," and *Gong* means "exercise" or "practice." In the West, people refer to this practice as creative visualization exercises. The book reported on cases of recoveries from chronic health conditions by using these thinking exercises, and I was drawn by their power.

Right away, I picked up the telephone to call the author, Master and Dr. Guo. I explained to him that I had a great interest in his work and asked if I could become his disciple. He told me, "At this moment, just be a student."

I was disappointed that Master Guo did not accept me as a disciple right away. You see, in China it has been the case for more than five thousand years that if you seriously want to learn the secrets of energy and spiritual healing, you have to become a disciple. It doesn't matter if you study with Buddhist, Taoist, Confucian, or other spiritual teachers. Disciples learn more secrets than ordinary students do.

"Disciple" means a committed student. "Master," a title of great honor, means a person who has been practicing in a field for many years, perhaps an entire lifetime, and has reached the "authority position" in that field. He or she receives respect from everyone in the field.

A disciple is a committed student who learns from the master and devotes himself or herself to study, research, and practice in that field. To be a disciple of a great master is a great honor. I am explaining this system because, in the West, many of you may not understand the relationship between master and disciple.

Let me continue my story with Master Guo. After he told me, "Just be a student now," he did not say when he would agree to accept me as a disciple. I felt disappointed, but at the same time I heard a very strong inner voice in my heart saying that I must become a disciple to learn the secrets of healing. I wanted to serve others, and I hoped Master Guo would consider my desire for service worthy enough to admit me as a disciple.

I was living in the Philippines at the time, practicing Chinese medicine and treating patients with Chinese herbs and acupuncture. I encouraged some of my friends and patients to make a healing journey to see Master Guo in China, although I could not go along with them at that time. People in the group had various unhealthy conditions, including arthritis, stomach ulcers, pain from gunshot wounds, and other ailments.

When the group returned to the Philippines one week later,

their health had improved so dramatically that I was shocked. My desire to become a disciple became even stronger. I telephoned Master Guo a few more times, but he kept saying, "Not yet. It's not the right time." Still, I did not give up. I called him again and again. I told him how interested I was in his work and that I wanted to learn his secrets.

Four months later, when I called Master Guo again, one of his five daughters answered the telephone and told me that Master Guo had gone thousands of miles away to Xinjiang province to teach Zhi Neng medicine. I asked for his telephone number there and called him that same day. He was surprised to hear from me. Again, I sincerely stated my request that he accept me as his disciple. He paused for a while on the phone, as if he was thinking about me or looking at me from a distance. Then he told me, "Wait until you get a letter from me." Right away, I felt there was hope.

I waited for ten days to get the letter. Finally, a half-page letter came. The opening salutation was "Disciple Zhi Gang." When I saw the word "Disciple," I was so touched that it brought tears to my eyes because I was so interested in the techniques and the healing results that Master Guo presented in his book. In the letter, he told me, "Study hard. Try your best to serve the people as a doctor. Don't forget your mother. Don't forget your country. Use the message of '3396815' [pronounced "sahn sahn joe lew bah yow woo" in Chinese] for communication between us." At that moment, I had no idea what "3396815" was or how to use it for communication with Master Guo. (I will offer this powerful communication and healing sound power technique to you in Chapter 8.)

Beginning in 1993, I started to receive serious training from Master Guo as a disciple. We began with the Open *San Jiao* (pronounced "sahn jow") body position: feet shoulder-width apart, toes gripping the earth, knees slightly bent, anus slightly contracted. He instructed me to place my right palm, facing upward, three inches above my navel and my left palm, facing upward, three inches below my navel and to hold this position for as long as I could in each practice session.

In the beginning, I could hold this fixed position for only one hour. My legs and body ached. After reporting to Master Guo, he told me, "Not enough! Do it more and longer!" After that, I did it for two hours. I felt warm, even hot, and I felt strong inner power. My body felt as if it were expanding. Then I reported to Master Guo again, and he said, "Not enough!" Next, I managed to do three hours. My whole body was boiling inside. Then I reported to him, and he said, "Still not enough!" I tried very hard to follow my master's instructions in order to win his approval. I practiced the position for longer and longer, until I could hold it for five hours at a time. Then Master Guo smiled and said, "This is your first step." (I will explain the Open *San Jiao* body power technique in Chapter 7.)

Next Master Guo taught me creative visualization to develop the most important energy centers in the body. These energy centers are called the Lower *Dan Tian* (pronounced "dahn tee-en"), the Snow Mountain Area, the Middle *Dan Tian* (also called the "Message Center"), the Upper *Dan Tian* (also called the "Third Eye"), and the *Zu Qiao* (pronounced "zoo chow"). (These five energy centers will be explained in detail in Chapter 11, where you will also find simple exercises for increasing their power.)

Master Guo also taught me how to develop the potential power of the brain. The left brain and right brain have different functions. The left brain is in charge of areas like logical thinking, mathematics, analysis, planning, and organization. The right brain is in charge of creative visualization, creativity, inspiration, Third Eye images, and so forth. The key to developing the potential power of the brain is to highly develop right-brain capabilities. To do this, Master Guo instructed me in the use of a special message and a special number code (which will be explained in Chapter 9).

Continuing to train with Master Guo, I became able to see bright light inside my Third Eye. Then I learned how to see images in the soul world. When I saw the images, I knew my Third Eye was opening.

Further training allowed me to open the Message Center to talk directly with God, other spiritual teachers and guides, angels, saints, Buddha, Jesus, Mary, and Muhammad, with everything in the universe. Because everything has a soul, communication is possible between all things in the universe. After you fully open your Message Center, which is located inside the center of the chest, you will be able to communicate with the souls of everything in the universe.

Moving to the next level, Master Guo started to train me how to see the image or energy field of the body's organs, looking for blockages. Many people who have opened their Third Eye can find blockages, but they may not know how to remove them. Finding the blockages is a great accomplishment, but removing them is even greater. Dr. Guo showed me a variety of techniques to remove blockages.

Then Master Guo trained me in Zhi Neng medicine energy massage and in Chinese herbs. He has created a new herb system called the Zhi Neng Medicine Herb System. This system uses only one hundred herbs, instead of the thousands of herbs in traditional Chinese medicine, to help heal all physical, mental, emotional, and spiritual illnesses.

After I mastered all the knowledge explained above, Master Guo said: "You are a good acupuncturist. You are the instructor at the World Health Organization's International Acupuncture Training Center in Beijing for physicians from all over the world. Let me guide you with a few points to improve your acupuncture capabilities." Then he told me secrets to make my acupuncture much more effective.

On October 12, 1994, after five years of devoted study of Zhi Neng medicine, Master Guo called me to his private study. I entered and saw him sitting in a full lotus position (see Figure 2). I bowed down to him and sat in a lotus position in front of him. We were both silent for several minutes. Then he started to talk.

"Zhi Gang, my lovely adopted son"—it was a great honor to be adopted in 1993 by Master Guo and Mrs. Guo, who have five daughters, as their only son—"and my first disciple, I give you the title of Zhi Neng Medicine Master and I give you this job: You are to be my representative to the West to spread Zhi Neng medicine to the whole world. This is the time for you to start your new journey in life."

I took my commission from Master Guo very seriously and investigated ways of spreading Zhi Neng medicine. I wrote a book entitled *Zhi Neng Medicine* in English and began my teaching journey in Canada. In 1997, I began to demonstrate qigong in the United States. I was invited to display my techniques at the World Congress on Qigong held in San Francisco. In that audience I was almost unknown, yet by the end of the conference I was honored and respected by many masters.

I share my story so that you will know how I found my masters on my journey and how I received the training I am passing on to you. My experience with Master Guo is the main story of my search for the secrets of healing. However, I have many stories from my studies with other teachers and masters who have helped me on my journey. I am profoundly grateful to them all.

I pass to you the essence of power healing: its four keys to gain power to heal your body, mind, and soul quickly. These techniques are in your hands NOW. Don't wait to practice them. Healing benefits will come to you right away.

"Thank you. Thank you. Thank you."

I close my seminars by repeating "Thank you" three times to show gratitude and honor. The first "Thank you" is to God. The second "Thank you" is to the members of your Heaven Team. Heaven Team refers to all the spirits in the spiritual world who love you, care for you and bless your life, including your spiritual teachers, healing angels, ascended masters, saints, guides, and ancestors. The third "Thank you" is to your own body, mind, and soul.

When the "Thank you" message is given in this book, I invite you to silently repeat "Thank you, thank you, thank you." In this small way, you can begin your study and practice of power healing: the four keys to energizing your body, mind, and spirit.

5

THE FOUR KEYS
TO POWER HEALING

As I have explained, many of the powerful self-healing techniques you're about to learn stem from Master and Dr. Guo's Zhi Neng medicine. In essence, I am his messenger and your guide.

I hesitate to reveal the power of power healing for fear that the stories will sound too good to be true. But you have already heard some powerful stories such as Paul's in Chapter 2. Let me also tell you about Robbie, a sixteen-year-old who had been deaf since birth. After just one healing session with me, he realized in a Burger King one afternoon that instead of lip-reading, he could actually hear the order taker for himself.

I know Western medicine can't cure deafness most of the time. But Western medicine is constantly discovering new things and learning ways to cure what was previously labeled incurable. So perhaps it's all a question of where you look for the answer or how you look at the problem to begin with.

That explains the results I was able to achieve with John Gray, whom you probably know from his best-seller *Men Are from Mars, Women Are from Venus*. I'll let him tell you how in his own words.

"I'd always been pretty healthy. But once I turned forty, my body changed, and a number of things started bothering me physically. No matter how spiritual I was, no matter how successful I was, no matter how much love I had in my relationships, there were still aches and pains that needed to be healed. But it took a much scarier problem to spur me to action.

"In 1992, an eye infection cost me most of the vision in my left eye. Suddenly I was legally blind in that eye. I couldn't even drive at night. Increasingly upset and depressed, I consulted sixteen or eighteen specialists, all of whom said they'd seen it in other people but could do nothing to help. There was no cure, they said. If it spread to both eyes, I'd be totally blind. Would it spread? They didn't know.

"Unwilling to give up, I began to seek alternative healers who might be able to help me. After six months of seeing acupuncturists and herbalists and, most important, taking time out from work in order to practice meditation techniques I'd learned in the past and changing my attitude about life, the vision in my left eye began to return. I knew a lot of that healing had to do with me and the power of my mind. I decided to find out more, especially since my eyesight, though seriously improved, had not been fully restored.

"Over the last nine years, my search for alternative healing and healers has taken me around the world twenty times. I've visited everyone from spiritual healers to chiropractors. But the energy healers impressed me the most. I believe that a lot of our illness comes from certain energy blocks, as well as attitudinal blocks like suppressed or negative emotion and mind-set. I've seen energy healers eliminate those blockages and provide people with exactly what their bodies needed to heal themselves. So whenever I would meet these healers, I would ask them to solve another problem that has come with age and take away the chronic pain in my feet.

Despite all their talent and the results I saw them achieving for others, no one was able to help me with that until I met Dr. Zhi Gang Sha. Although I had traveled the world in search of healers, I would meet this master in the San Francisco Bay Area, where I live.

"As an avid seeker of alternative health solutions, I'd gone to the 2000 Whole Life Expo. Dr. Sha's credentials looked good to me on paper, so I made a point of seeking him out. When I got there, he was preparing to do a healing demonstration in front of a live audience. He asked for a volunteer, and I raised my hand. I went up to the front, and he did a short healing on the one foot that was really bothering me. Five minutes later, the pain was gone. Completely gone. A week later, when the pain had not returned, I asked him to treat my other foot. That was a year ago, and the pain has yet to return in either foot.

"Figuring that I had nothing to lose, I asked him to treat my allergies next. All my life I've suffered miserably from hay fever, and just as miserably from the various drugs I would take to control my allergies. I couldn't stand the intense side effects, which for me included drowsiness, irritability, and discomfort. After seven sessions with Dr. Sha and his assistants, all my symptoms simply disappeared. For the rest of the season I was allergy free. (I'm waiting to find out how I fare this year.) In addition, with a single exception, I haven't even suffered from colds or the flu, both of which I used to get all the time."

John Gray praises my healing abilities, for which I'm very grateful. But he worked hard to help himself. And in so doing, a number of "incurable" problems were suddenly reversed.

"Don't try this at home" warn so many television programs. But that's just what I want you to do. The healer is within you. You can do it!

My techniques are very simple, practical, and easy to implement. Most important, they work.

As you know, the secret to triggering your self-healing system lies in balancing the transformation between matter inside cells and energy outside cells. That needs to happen on the three equally important levels of the body, the mind, and the soul.

The four keys to power healing, for balancing and boosting energy, are body power, sound power, mind power, and soul power. Let me introduce them briefly.

BODY POWER

Body power techniques include special hand, standing, and sitting positions that can help you heal your body, mind, and soul by opening your energy and communication channels. These techniques will help you:

- Gain power and energy in your internal organs
- Develop the power of your energy centers, a key to increasing immunity and stamina
- Heal your body, mind, and soul by promoting energy flow in your meridians (the energy pathways)
- Increase the effectiveness of your immune system to prevent illness
- Improve the quality of your life
- Prolong your life
- Open your Message Center, the energy center that allows you to talk directly with your mind, the organs and cells in your body, God (whatever your belief system may be), your Heaven Team (which includes all your spiritual teachers and guides, angels, archangels, ascended masters, saints, ancestors, and everyone else in the spiritual world who loves you,

cares for you, and helps you on your spiritual and life journeys), and your own soul

- Open your Third Eye (the seat of your ability to see images
  of the spiritual world and energy or energy blockages in the
  body) so that you can see the soul world and share love, care,
  and compassion with your Heaven Team and God

- Enlighten your spiritual journey

SOUND POWER

Practitioners in the East have long used mantras, repeated phrases
or series of sounds, in a particular and sustained way.

Each mantra has its own message. Some mantras have a special
message for healing, developing energy, or opening the Third
Eye. Others have a special message for opening your Message
Center (to converse directly with God and your Heaven Team) or
blessing or protecting your life. Indeed, a powerful mantra may
include many such special messages.

Every mantra also has a special sound. That sound vibrates different parts of the body and carries special energy. As such, it can
be used for healing, blessing, protecting, and improving the quality of your cells, organs, body, mind, and soul.

When you practice a mantra, you do not practice only one
time. You do not practice only a few times. When you chant a
mantra, you should practice for at least ten to fifteen minutes,
and perhaps as much as a half hour, an hour, or even many hours.
Why? Suppose, for example, that you chant a mantra to remove
an energy blockage at the cellular level. The power of the mantra
can do this. The special message and the special sound of the
mantra will stimulate the vibration of the cells and organs. The

mantra will balance the transformation between the matter inside the cells and the energy outside the cells. This balance takes time to be accomplished. That's why one of the keys to successful mantra practice is repetition, saying the mantra over and over and over and over.

The sound power technique of chanting mantras and other special healing sounds will help you:

- Gain energy and stamina for your body, mind, and soul

- Strengthen your immune system

- Heal and balance yourself physically, emotionally, mentally, and spiritually

- Purify your heart and soul

- Improve the cellular condition of your body

- Share love, care, compassion, sincerity, honesty, and kindness with millions of people at the same time

- Get blessings for the success of your work and the harmony of your relationships and for the promotion of safety and peace in your life

- Increase your healing power

- Develop the potential capabilities of your body, mind, and soul, such as opening your Message Center

- Clean your karma

- Become enlightened and fulfilled on your spiritual journey

- Gain inspiration from the soul world to develop your intelligence and the wisdom of your body, mind, and soul

- Understand deeply the secrets, principles, and laws of the universe and human beings

MIND POWER

Creative visualization can develop the brain and heal body, mind, and soul. Brain researchers explain we have about fifteen billion brain cells. In our entire life, we use only 10 percent of our brain cells. I call the unused 90 percent "potential" brain cells. Awakening and developing the potential power of those dormant brain cells should be a goal for every person who wants to develop his or her mind. Therein lies a significant portion of your power to self-heal.

SOUL POWER

Mind over matter is not enough, however. Soul over matter is much more powerful. Soul power is soul healing, message healing, and soul communication.

Though you may not realize it, more and more of you are searching for soul knowledge and soul enlightenment. More and more of you want to know the purpose of life. Why do some of you feel you have no direction? Feel irritable? Feel depressed? You may not be aware that your irritability and depression are rooted in issues of your soul. You may be successful and wealthy, but your soul may not be happy. If you have happiness, health, personal satisfaction, and fulfilling work, your soul will be happy and you will feel that God and heaven are blessing you.

After more than thirty years of studying traditional Chinese arts and medicine, Western medicine, different religions, and other spiritual studies and philosophies, I've come to understand that soul power is the number-one issue in the whole world and the most important power-healing technique I can share with you. Why? Because it's one of the most important issues in a human being's life. Soul affects personal health, happiness, and business success. In short, soul is the essence of life.

How the Four Keys Work Together

You'll soon see how practical and profound these four keys are to power healing. But I want you to understand how simple they are to use, how powerful they are when used together, and how quickly they can bring healing results.

During a self-healing workshop I was leading not long ago, I asked whether anyone was suffering from back pain. Many people quickly raised their hands. I chose one person, a man named Tony, to come forward. Then I began to show him how to self-heal.

First I introduced him to the notion of body power, the special hand, sitting, and standing positions that stimulate cellular vibration, promote energy flow, and remove energy blockages. Tony's back pain meant that there was an energy blockage in his back.

"Please stand in front of me," I said to Tony. "This is the basic standing position. You will use it many times. Stand with your feet shoulder-width apart, bend your knees slightly, keep your back straight, and keep your body relaxed." In a moment, Tony was comfortable. "Tony, I am going teach you the One Hand Near, One Hand Far Self-Healing Method. Tony, use your right hand as the near hand and place it behind your back. Use your fingertips to point to the painful area. Keep your near hand 4 to 8 inches away from your body. Now use your left hand as the far hand. Place it 12 to 20 inches away from the front of your lower abdomen, with your palm facing your body." Tony shifted his weight back and forth and found a comfortable place for his hands.

Then I began to teach Tony about sound power, which uses healing mantras and special healing sounds. These sounds promote energy flow and remove energy blockages. I said to Tony, "Now chant one sound with me: Hoooonnnngggg, hoooonnnngggg, hoooonnnngggg, hoooonnnngggg." *Hong* vibrates and stimulates cellular vibration in the lower back.

Now Tony was ready to learn about mind power, which utilizes creative visualization to promote healing. I suggested to Tony: "Keep your hands and body in the same position. Continue to chant '*Hong, hong, hong, hong.*' Repeat this over and over. At the same time, visualize the brightest light you can radiating in your painful lower back area."

Tony was comfortable, smiling and enjoying the exercise, when I introduced the fourth technique, soul power. "Everybody has a soul. Every part of the body has a soul. Your lower back has a soul also, and you can communicate directly with your lower back," I told Tony. "Say these words to your lower back: 'I love my lower back. I request the soul of my lower back to heal my lower back. My lower back is vibrating. Energy flows in my lower back perfectly.' Visualize light continuously radiating in your painful lower back area and say, 'Light, light, light, light . . . ' Say '*Hao, hao, hao*' (pronounced 'how'), which means 'Get well,' 'Get stronger.' Then say 'Thank you, thank you, thank you.'"

The audience watched intently as Tony applied himself to these four techniques simultaneously. They were amazed when Tony turned and exclaimed how much relief he felt in his lower back. Tony came back to another of my workshops the next month to thank me because his back pain had not returned.

MESSAGE THEORY

"I don't understand how all this works," I hear you saying. "What's all that talking to your body and your soul about anyway?" Let me add to the explanation.

Physics in the West has studied the concepts of matter and energy for millennia. To most people, matter is composed of particles that are tangible and specific in a place. Energy, on the other hand, is composed of waves that are less tangible and spread out.

In the Matter-Energy Message Theory of Zhi Neng medicine, message is the link—the communication line—between matter and energy. Since all messages communicate with each other in the universe, this link between energy and matter is not a one-way communication; it can be a two-way or a many-way communication. (Western scientific theory may support this notion. Some physicists now talk of the connection between matter, thought, and information. Cellular biologists are developing a clear biochemical understanding of cellular communication at the molecular level.)

The four power-healing techniques (body, sound, mind, and soul power) are all messages that work at the cellular level to balance the transformation between the matter inside the cells and the energy outside the cells. Similarly, all herbs, vitamins, and other remedies carry their own messages. Proper use of these messages will bring good healing results because they promote *chi* flow. They all balance the transformation between the matter inside the cells and the energy outside the cells at the cellular level. That is why message is the key to helping people become healthy, happy, nourished, satisfied, and enlightened.

However strange it may sound to you right now, the four power-healing techniques provide a practical way to improve your health. As with John Gray, they may even give you a way to solve those "incurable" problems of your own. Of course you will have to come to terms with all these new ideas in your own way. But perhaps Mary Ellen's story—and that of her friend Jan—will help you do that.

"As far back as the early 1970s, as a nursing student, I recall attending a lecture given by a doctor who spent a number of years living and working in China. This was my first exposure to energy in the body, energy pathways, and acupuncture. I filed this away as an intriguing notion in health care.

"After working about ten years in different medical disciplines, I came to a crossroads. I wanted to explore natural healing. I became a massage therapist as well as a practitioner of Japanese acupressure. Now I had an opportunity, in my own clinic, to try this energy work. I was amazed at the results my patients were reporting. At this point I had to know more about energy. In the material I read, one word came up frequently and that was qigong, an energy healing exercise system. How could these masters from China, using their hands in specific poses, create such healing?

"My husband and I moved to the West Coast in search of a qigong master to teach me how to heal this way. Meeting Dr. Sha was a thrilling experience. I knew immediately that he was beyond a qigong master. I knew that he would teach me how to build, manipulate, move, stimulate, and heal with energy.

"Energy is not only elusive, but it also manifests itself in many forms such as sound, light, soul, and mind energy. Also, specific hand positions can direct and intensify its effects on the body. It is my personal belief that we are energy beings encased in a physical body, so it makes great sense to me that, if we are ailing in our physical beings, we have the ability and power to balance and heal ourselves through these energy forms and techniques. It was my goal to learn as much about energy as I could, because it was my personal desire to move beyond physical manipulation, as in massage and acupressure, and heal without touching people, using energy flow only.

"Not long ago, I was blessed with such a healing opportunity. A dear friend, Jan, an athlete, suffered an injury to her right leg called shin splints. This is an extremely painful condition common to runners. The pain radiates down the lower leg and, depending on the severity of the injury, the person may not be able to bear weight on the leg. With my medical background, I understood the conventional method of treatment. Jan used crutches for a short time, ingested copious amounts of pain-killers and anti-inflammatories, and received physiotherapy treatments. After a year she was still unable to resume her power walking and could only walk for short periods before the pain returned.

"Jan came to visit my husband and me before she was to see an orthopedic surgeon. Still unable to walk without pain, she agreed to let me try to help. She sat comfortably in a chair and I positioned myself in front of her. I began with my arm outstretched and my fingertips pointing to Jan's shin and, more specifically, to where she felt the pain. Next, I chanted the natural sound of the number 11 (pronounced "shuh-ee" in Chinese) which stimulates cellular vibration in the legs and arms. I also asked Jan to repeat "shuh-ee" so that she could participate actively in the healing. Next was the creative visualization of a very bright white light radiating up and down her shin and, with all these techniques in place, I asked the healing spirits to bless my friend. After only three to four minutes, I knew from within myself that the healing was complete. I remember Jan saying, 'Is that all?' with utter disbelief that anything had happened.

"Realizing that Jan couldn't tolerate much walking, we had planned our day with a little sightseeing that required minimal walking. The day progressed with no complaint of leg pain from Jan. While we were having dinner, we asked how her leg felt. Our question prompted her to think about her leg for the first time after the healing that morning. She started to cry with the realization that she did not have any more pain and, with all the walking we did, she normally would have been in agony by this time.

"The next morning, she got up with no pain and decided to try to go for an hour-long power walk. I taught her another chant to use while walking in order to boost her energy and enhance her healing. The chant was the special healing number '3396815' ('sahn sahn joe lew bah yow woo'), which gives the body an internal energy massage and is a key to energy development. Jan successfully completed her power walk and, after returning, still had no pain. Since then, Jan has walked regularly, sometimes power walking for an hour, twice a day, with no further discomfort. I am truly humble and grateful to have been able to help my friend using these simple techniques."

The four keys to power healing I've just introduced to you will give you the power to improve your health, your habits, and your life. The simple, quick, and effective techniques you'll learn will vitalize self-healing, just as eating food, drinking water, and breathing air vitalize life itself. Whether you use them in conjunction with any and all conventional medical practices or alternative health methods or on their own, they will help you discover your relationship with your own health. You will come to know—and love—the healer within you.

6

THE JOY OF SELF-HEALING

I t's hard to believe that this kind of natural, noninvasive healing can work so quickly to effect physical changes that can be so profound. But it does, as a number of studies will show you.

BLOOD CELL ANALYSIS

Jill and Daniel are certified microscopists who analyze live blood cells. They perform this analysis by placing a drop of blood from the client's fingertip on a cover slip, which is promptly covered by a glass slide to keep the blood from drying out. The slide is then viewed at high magnification on a compound microscope that projects the image on a video monitor. In this way, the quality of a person's health at the cellular level is revealed. Rounded, symmetrical red cells that are all about the same size and separated from each other, for example, show that the blood is able to provide the oxygen necessary to all the different parts of the body.

The process provides not only current information about a person's state of health, but also information about patterns that could cause trouble in the future. Pathologies, for example, appear in the blood sometimes years before they manifest themselves as illness.

In connection with their work, Daniel and Jill became curious about energy healing because of its concern with moving energy in and out of cells. So in February 2001 they attended a seminar on the topic. That's where they met me.

"Before we saw Dr. Sha's work we were a little skeptical about the concept of healing energy," says Daniel. "However, we were pleasantly surprised by Dr. Sha's passion and energy. He grabbed the attention of everyone in the room."

Of course, that didn't mitigate their skepticism, which they fully expected to justify when they proposed testing participants in a cancer recovery program I led in conjunction with John Gray (who has himself become a powerful healer) to see what—if any—effects the healing would have on the patients' blood. I'll let Daniel and Jill tell you what they found in their own words:

"The following is our findings on performing the live blood cell analysis before and after the energy healing. We were very careful in taking several blood samples to obtain a true reading and to eliminate operator error. We viewed the blood before the healing. We saw multiple indications of disorganized red blood cells clumping and sticking together and fibrin spicules (seen as little black lines) in the blood, which indicates liver or bowel stress.

"Participants then went through the healing with Dr. Sha. After the healing, they sat and waited twenty minutes. Then we tested the participants again. In many cases we saw amazing results in the blood.

"One of the remarkable results was that red blood cells went from sticking together to moving freely. This is usually only seen when a person drinks a large amount of water over a period of several hours, since a primary reason for red blood cells to stick together is dehydration.

"In short, the energy work affected the blood in a positive fashion. We saw signs of the blood going from an unbalanced state to a more balanced state after a single healing session, changes that would normally take days, if not weeks, of dietary change to produce."

BODY-CHEMISTRY ASSESSMENT

Joan Kasich—a natural health consultant and herb specialist from Moraga, California, who's certified in the areas of nutrition, herbology, live and dry blood cell analysis, and body-chemistry assessment—decided to conduct a body-chemistry assessment on the cancer recovery program participants. By analyzing their urine and their saliva first in November 2000 and then two months later in January 2001, she would see whether the healing sessions had made a statistically significant improvement in the chemistry of the participants' bodies.

Results from the seventeen individuals who completed both the before and after tests were significant. "When initially tested, every single person showed an unbalanced pH level," says Kasich. "When your pH level is out of balance (which usually happens because of stress, poor nutrition, or toxins), the body has to borrow minerals like calcium, sodium, potassium, and magnesium from the vital organs and bones to buffer acid caused by undigested proteins and safely remove it from the body. I believe this demineralization process, which throws the pH level further out of balance, causes disease. As the pH level nears the target 6.4 level, the body stops losing minerals, thereby allowing the organs to absorb more nutrition. Balance the pH and your body will heal itself of any of the physical ailments that plague you, whether allergies, skin eruptions, joint problems, or cancer."

After less than ten weeks, 59 percent of those tested by Kasich showed significant improvement in their pH levels. (Three months later, one of the participants who had shown remarkable improvement in her pH level would even announce that a recent liver scan no longer revealed any traces of cancer.) Among those participants tested, 65 percent showed marked improvement in their digestion, a critical component of wellness.

"What the chemistries do not reflect is the overall shift I saw in people's faces and behavior as the project unfolded," says Kasich. "I noticed more brightness in people's eyes, more color in their cheeks, more animation. As the project went on, the stamina of most of the participants seemed to increase. And I saw a general increase in the happiness of the group. Happiness is health."

As Kasich points out, the power healing she witnessed was taking place on an emotional level as well as on a physical level. Before any of the physical changes could take place, a shift in attitude had to occur. In short, the participants had to believe that they could effect a change in their health.

MOTIVATION

But let's face it—belief is not enough. New Age consciousness notwithstanding, neither are affirmations. You must actively seek and then make a new reality, first by accessing the energy of desire. If you're already well, you'll experience no desire to get healthy. If you're unwell, then you first have to start with the realization of where you are, then generate the desire and will to leave it behind, as in: "I need help. I want help. I want to get healed, and I'm willing to do something about it."

That last point is just as important as the first. You can think, "My body's getting better and better" or "Every day I wake up, my life is getting better and better," and that's great. But if that's all you're doing, it's not going to have an effect. If you're lucky, it will simply keep you where you are. All too often, however, if we're not doing anything to make things better, they just get worse.

Affirmations simply aren't enough without action. I remember one woman in her thirties whose life had steadily gone from fair to poor. Her career as a freelance television producer was slowly drying up. Though she yearned to be married, she'd had no romantic attachments for several years. But instead of doing something to change all that, she sat in her apartment surrounded by positive sayings written out on Post-Its, which were stuck on everything from her computer to her refrigerator. "The universe will provide," she routinely asserted when asked why she wasn't pursuing other options more actively. The universe, however, only provides to those who take action to get what they want.

Ultimately, you have to help yourself. That sense of affirmation is just the start of your healing, of getting blockages released and your energy flowing again. Then you must take the initiative to solve your problem. Just making that decision alone will positively impact your health, because that sends a message to your body and your brain that you have the power to change your situation. Feeling hope instead of despair, control instead of helplessness, will start to unblock your energy. But that's just the beginning. You have to be willing to keep doing the work, to stay the course.

Desire is a big part of what makes healing happen. You have to really want it. Increased desire creates more motivation and more energy to re-create and heal yourself. But you need to participate in that healing. If you depend on the notion that someone else is ultimately going to do the job for you, your own efforts will be subverted. If, on the other hand, you assume that you can learn to self-heal and then put forth effort, you will get results.

The Chinese tell a story about a healer who sat on top of a mountain where the sick and the weak would struggle to reach him and be cured. "Why don't you go down to the town to heal the people?" he was asked. "The really sick people can't get up here, and only those who finally do make it up benefit."

The healer refused. "Unless they make the trek up here, they're not ready for the healing," he replied.

It's one thing to believe that you will be healed, but another to make some sacrifices to get there. In other words, intention plus appropriate action equal results. It all starts and ends with you. You must put in the time and the energy. Every time you're climbing that mountain to get healed and your body tells you, "I don't want to do this" and your mind tells you, "I don't want to do this," you have to come back and say, "but I want to get healed." And then push ahead—do it anyway.

That's the bottom line. No matter what's bothering you, you want to get healed. So you do what it takes.

That's not always easy in our society. "Today, our appetites have been whetted with quick fixes, so much so that our quest for diagnostic gadgets and miracle drugs has almost overcome common sense. We expect that surgical acumen will be enough to save us and if not, the next remarkable scientific discovery will," writes Herbert Benson, M.D., in his book *The Relaxation Response.* "Although mind/body therapies have been proven effective for the vast majority of everyday medical problems, we are still far more apt to run to our medicine cabinet to relieve aches and pains than to consider relaxation or stress-management techniques."[1]

We are also prone to judge self-healing's effectiveness way too quickly. It's crazy. People who have hypertension take medicine their whole lives without a single complaint. Yet with self-healing, they try once or twice and then give up, saying that nothing happened when they don't see any change. That's not fair.

Practicing the self-healing methods you're about to learn should become a routine part of your daily life. These power-healing techniques are just as important for self-healing as food, water, and air are for life.

This is the ultimate system of regaining control over your own life, over yourself. And these days that's downright critical. "Change is more accelerated than it's ever been in the world outside us," says John Gray, whose book *Practical Miracles for Mars and Venus* deals with that very topic, providing nine guiding principles that can help you adjust to life's challenges. "If we don't use our ability to change quickly on the inside, we will experience increasingly more stress from that external revolution."

Amazingly, however, most of us have no idea how much control we actually do have over our own health. Studies, for example, have shown that humans can successfully lower their blood pressure simply by meditating or thinking relaxing thoughts.[2] Even monkeys can be trained to control their blood pressure without medications. Of course, not all physical conditions respond this readily. But even when we can't control what happens to us, we can control our reactions—which will influence what happens next.

"This sounds like a lot of hard work," I hear you say. That's where you're wrong. Self-healing does take motivation, determination, and persistence. But it's not a negative thing. To the contrary. Self-healing is joyful, fun. It's talking, singing, dancing. It's focusing on life plans instead of illness, on how to get the most from your life as you do all you can to renew and revitalize it.

Of course, it doesn't always seem that way at first.

"You feel an overwhelming and unforgettable sense of shock when you are told you have cancer," writes Jackie, a woman in her early forties. "And you're especially shocked when your body feels fine.

"Physically I felt better then ever, but emotionally I never felt worse. Being a writer, television producer, and sought-after speaker on social change and self-esteem issues, I had no time to be sick. Ironically, I was just finishing production on a television show for PBS called 'Healthy Living,' all about the connection between health and happiness.

"That definitely got my attention. 'Healthy Living' and I had cancer! I'd always prided myself on my health. I had to stop and wonder if I had not been living a lie. Here I had been teaching exactly what I needed to learn the most: the keys to health, happiness, and self-esteem. My spirit was shaken to its core.

"Many things had gone wrong. But first let me tell you there is a miracle in this story. According to *Newsweek,* 84 percent of us believe in miracles and 42 percent of us have experienced one. Well, I am one of the 42 percent, thanks to my brother.

"Six months prior to my diagnosis, my professional life started to fall apart. I had some devastating setbacks. A television series I'd pitched got picked up—by a producer who turned out to be a three-time convicted felon. John F. Kennedy, Jr., agreed to be our speaker at a fund-raiser we were having—less than a month after the contracts were signed he was killed. After co-authoring several best-selling books, my partner and I had a nasty breakup. I had created and carried out a special humanitarian mission to Macedonia during the Kosovo war by bringing thirty-five clown doctors, medical supplies, toys, balloons, beanie babies, and some great entertainment and love in the form of Patch Adams, M.D., to the 143,000 refugees and children living in the deplorable refugee camps. A live satellite global feed on Fox News was scheduled with a news team from England. What a great opportunity to show direct action and love in action! That story was suddenly scrapped for a border-massacre headline story. You know, if it bleeds, it leads. Although I was terribly moved by the joy and laughter on the faces of the kids and parents whose lives we had touched in the camps, I still felt like I had not done enough.

Everything good seemed to manifest, only to deconstruct, disintegrate, or derail.

"I began to feel I couldn't do anything. I felt that my life did not matter. I started to think about death. Two very close and dear friends had died in these six months too. I wondered about joining them. Maybe I could do more from the other side. I just did not feel I could find a place or a project that could receive my love and what I had to offer. I questioned whether I was good enough. But at least I had my health. Or so I thought.

"Years ago, my brother and I had a big falling out. Our splintered relationship started to weigh on me more and more heavily. I really suffered his loss. For years I had been meditating and looking at many spiritual practices. I knew about the power of prayer, so I prayed to God to heal our relationship. Just one month later the phone rang. He needed surgery and wanted me to come to Baltimore and take care of him.

"I was of course terribly worried, but also deeply heartened to hear him asking for me. I later learned that he had gone on vacation to go deep-sea fishing with some friends. The friends had an emergency and had to cancel. Not wanting to go alone, my brother invited a perfect stranger who just happened to be vacationing next door. They were out on the high seas when this perfect stranger, who turned out to be a foot doctor, happened to notice my brother's ailing toe and ordered him to have blood tests prior to taking some medicine he insisted on prescribing.

"The blood tests showed severe anemia, which is a sign of iron deficiency, certain illnesses and diseases, or internal bleeding. The battery of tests that was immediately ordered up revealed a golf ball–sized tumor in his colon.

"My brother had never felt better, so the tumor diagnosis was a shock. But not as big a shock as the news the surgeon gave us in the waiting room outside the O.R.: the tumor was malignant and I needed to be tested immediately for the same thing.

"To prove I was healthy, I dutifully submitted to a round of tests. Much to my shock and horror, I was diagnosed with the same thing. So less than a month after my brother's surgery and recovery, I had surgery too. Imagine two people so far apart being brought together over what appeared to be a tragedy. There is no stronger bond than the bond you form with someone who shares a trauma or similar tragedy. But the tragedy turned into an out-and-out miracle. The doctor said that we had both found these cancers so early that no follow-up treatment was needed. On every level what had looked like a disaster turned into a blessing.

"I did not realize I was in store for another brush with death. After healing with my brother, I returned home and went back to work. During a meeting, I suddenly began to suffer from horrible abdominal pains that sent me straight to the doctor. He performed a uterine biopsy, which led to a series of tests and surgeries.

"The words that you have cancer do not sound any better the second time, especially when it's the second time in four months. However, when the oncologist broke the news, adding that a number of surgeries would be required to find out how extensive the cancer was, I happened to glance over at his bookshelf where I spotted a clown doctor figurine. I flashed on Patch Adams telling me how needed and necessary I was, and I knew that, somehow, I would again be fine. I immediately stood up. 'Wow, this is a miracle!' I announced to the doctor. 'I'm going to be cured of cancer twice in the same year.'

"Thank God working as a clown doctor with Patch had taught me how healing humor is. Deciding that I would use humor—in addition to prayer—to help beat this cancer, I painted green four-leaf clovers all over my legs before a surgery that had been scheduled for St. Patrick's Day. They complemented the green wig and bright green dress I wore to the hospital quite nicely. In the operating suite, where all those scheduled for surgery wait so nervously, I told a series of jokes—the kind that make you cry from laughing so hard—that a friend had e-mailed me. Smiles and laughter everywhere. When I woke up in the recovery room, I couldn't help but smile upon noticing the four-leaf clovers I still had on my legs. And, you know, I really felt great, probably because of all the laughter that day.

"Before my laproscopic hysterectomy, I planned a surprise going-away party for my malignant uterus in the waiting room just outside the O.R. We had balloons, clowns, music, presents, and surprises for the hospital staff, my family, and friends. You would have never guessed you were in a hospital. I came through the surgery fine and surprised the doctors by being out of bed and walking very shortly thereafter. After eight weeks of daily radiation treatment I was released by my doctors to return to work.

"Now, one would think that I would be on top of the world, elated to be alive and ready to make every moment count, not knowing how much longer I had on this earth. Well, I guess you could say I was suffering from a bit of post-traumatic stress disorder. I became terrified about a recurrence. I feared death, but I also feared life. I couldn't move. I was stuck. Convinced that my lifestyle and emotional reactions to my work and all those work-related disappointments had led to my illness, I was afraid to work again and engage in any relationships that might become toxic. I knew that stress, failure, unfulfilled dreams, desires, and hopes, not being able to effect change and produce results, and pushing hard against something you cannot move all can create cancer. Not finding ways to be of service can create stress too, but I was afraid to try. I was hibernating and in isolation. That is when I met Dr. Sha and was introduced to his self-healing techniques.

"If you ask me, the recovery period after you finish with surgery and treatment are the most critical times. That is when you can successfully live and get back into life, or just get sick again and die. Although a certain amount of adrenaline gets you through the surgery and treatments, you don't have that during your recovery. The power of self-healing, of knowing I could help myself, is what propelled me back into action. Although I was very rusty, things started to flow. I chanted. I moved. I sang. I danced. I worked to heal others. And I laughed as I healed myself."

Jackie literally transformed herself from a woman who couldn't even drag herself off the couch to a bundle of energy who worked sixteen hours a day, wore a nonstop smile, and looked like the health-and-vitality poster girl.

"She's sick?" one man asked after meeting her. "She can't be. She positively glows."

He was right.

"I'm happy to report my last tests showed I am cancer free," says Jackie. "My brother and I talk nearly every day. I am deeply grateful and totally convinced that joy in healing makes all the difference."

As Jackie discovered, the impact resulting from this joyous—and joyful—power healing can be life-changing. As you are about to see, however, the techniques are quite simple.

7

BODY POWER

Why do millions of practitioners of qigong, Buddhism, Taoism, Confucianism, tai chi, and other healing arts practice body power techniques daily? Because they get the job done.

There are thousands of these techniques that can be used to gain energy and heal the body, mind, and soul—far too many to discuss all of them here. I will only introduce you to four, but they'll be enough to enhance your life. I hope that you will continue to use any body-related power techniques you may have learned before this, in addition to those you will learn from this book. They all will work for you.

Body power techniques are special hand and body positions that make energy flow by using different energy fields. Whether healers realize this or not, all healing disciplines, whatever philosophy lies behind them and wherever they come from, work at the cellular level to heal. Let me remind you what we're talking about here: *chi,* the energy that radiates from your cells and organs. After all, in traditional Chinese medicine, *chi* means "vital energy" and "life force"—so you've got to have good *chi* inside and out if you want a healthy, balanced, and happy life.

As you know, *chi* is the energy that is transformed from matter inside the cells and inside the organs. This energy is given different names, depending on which organ or part of the body the *chi* radiates out from. *Chi* that radiates out from the heart, for example, is named heart *chi*. *Chi* that radiates out from the kidneys is called kidney *chi*, and *chi* that radiates out from the brain is called brain *chi*. Although each organ, indeed each part of the body, has its own *chi* name, they are all part of the body's single energy system. So for the system to be in balance, all the organs must breathe out and breathe in the proper amount of energy.

When the *chi* of the different organs radiates out in a harmonious way, you have good health. When any organ vibrates too much or too little from bacterial or other infections or from emotional imbalance and stress, then the *chi* of the organs will radiate out in a disharmonious way and sickness will occur.

If we expand on this concept of one single life energy in the body, we can hypothesize that there's only one *chi* in the universe. When the sun radiates energy, we enjoy the sunshine. The *chi* radiating out from the sun is named the *chi* of the sun. When you sit down by a lake at night with your girlfriend or boyfriend, you feel the love, peace, and harmony of the lake and the moon. The *chi* radiating out from the lake is named the *chi* of the lake. The *chi* radiating out from the moon is named the *chi* of the moon. When you go to the pyramids in Egypt, you feel the *chi* of the pyramids. When you go to the Great Wall of China, you feel the *chi*, or energy, of the Great Wall. When you stand beside the Pacific Ocean, your feel your chest expand as you breathe in the moist air and feel the *chi* of the ocean. When you go to the Amazon rain forest, you feel the *chi* of the Amazon rain forest.

This discussion about *chi* can be summarized in one sentence: *chi* is the energy radiating out from matter. But there is also *chi* in personal names and in business names. Your name has its own *chi.* So does the name of your company, of any business. Your health, happiness, and success are closely related to both your personal name and your business name. If your business isn't successful, please be aware that the name of your business may not be proper. Every business name has its own *chi* and message. To improve your business, you must find out its proper and blessed name.

To change your life, you must find out your own proper and blessed name. Some people have names that carry unhealthy and unpleasant *chi* and messages. Those people feel unfulfilled. They cannot attain success and happiness. Power-healing techniques, however, can train you to fully open your Message Center in order to read the *chi* and message of your personal name and business name. You'll learn these techniques later on. Once you develop the ability to communicate with the spiritual world, you can also receive guidance in changing your personal and business names. Over the last ten years, I have personally trained many people to develop these capabilities.

Let's take this one step further. People in the West are becoming more and more interested in feng shui (pronounced "fung shway"). What's that? Feng shui is the ancient Chinese philosophy and practice of determining the energy and message inside and outside the house, business office, and surrounding areas. When a woman learns the principles of feng shui from a book or a workshop, for example, she may move her bed around and change the position of the tables, desks, chairs, and lamps. "What are you doing?" asks her husband. "I am making our home more pleasant," she replies. In fact, she is allowing the energy in her home to circulate more freely.

Everything in a house radiates *chi,* or energy. If the furniture blocks the *chi* flow in a room, it will affect your health. The furniture inside a business office must also be placed in a proper way.

The environment surrounding the house or office, including buildings, roads, trees, mountains, gardens, and water, also affects the health of the occupants and the success of the business.

If the *chi* of your home or office is·unbalanced, it will affect your health and business. Moving the furniture, plants, and mirrors in and around your house and office can promote health, happiness, and success. If you feel that the furnishings and decorations are not properly placed, then consult a feng shui master to determine the best arrangement. If you do, your health and your business will improve.

If you cannot find a feng shui master, let me teach you a simple way to change the energy in your bedroom. If you cannot sleep well at night, change the direction of your bed and see whether that makes any difference to your sleep. Move your bed around a few more times to find the best position for a good night's sleep.

Next, let me teach you a simple technique that will allow you to improve the feng shui of your home or office. Go into any room of your house or office and sit down. Totally relax your body. Calm your mind. Close your eyes slightly. Try to get a feeling for that room. Do you feel peace, comfort, and joy? Or do you feel irritable, uncomfortable, and unpleasant? Peace, comfort, and joy tell you that the *chi* and messages of that room are in harmony. In other words, that room has good feng shui. Irritability, discomfort, and unpleasantness tell you that the *chi* and messages of that room are not in harmony. In other words, that room does not have good feng shui. A change is necessary.

One of the most important elements for good feng shui in a home or office is to have enough space around the furniture. This will allow *chi* to flow smoothly. After you make some changes to improve the *chi* flow, use the same knowledge and techniques to feel the new energy flow in the environment.

In my years of practice, I have seen many who suffer from chronic pain and illness. They see doctors and all kinds of healers, but they do not realize that their home, office, business location, or hometown is affecting their health. Some people who cannot tolerate cold weather move to the Arizona desert in the winter and feel better. Some people with asthma move to another city and get well. Some people who do not have asthma move to another city and get asthma, because the *chi*, or energy, in the new city is inappropriate for their health. Why? Because the *chi* of the area or something in the area affects health. Therefore, when you get sick, see your doctor or healer, but don't forget that the *chi* and the messages of the environment may be affecting your health.

Chi also affects the health and harmony of your relationships. Although everybody radiates *chi*, each person's *chi* carries a different message. *Chi* has different frequencies. If the *chi* between friends matches, then the friendship is harmonious. If the *chi* between friends does not match, then the friendship is not harmonious. If the *chi* between a man and a woman is harmonious, then they feel happy. If the *chi* is not in harmony, they are not happy.

The practice of the power-healing techniques you're about to learn can improve the *chi* of the body at the cellular level and at the organ level. Beyond that, it can improve the capabilities of your mind and soul. Then your view of the world and of relationships will change. You can forgive more easily. You will take more responsibility for your own mistakes instead of blaming others. Your relationships with the world will be more harmonious.

"My boss is very detail-oriented and driven," writes Andrew, an expert in environmental issues and public policy. "He has a way of making you very nervous, especially if you are under the least bit of stress. Sometimes my stomach will tie up in knots and I will have incredible anxiety attacks fearing that I will not be able to get all the work done in time and with the precision and detail he demands. Not only do I have to worry about the detail work, we have all these political relationships and very sensitive strategic alliances to manage.

"Right before heading off to give a lecture at a conference in Florida, I had a talk with the head of an organization with which we had one of our sensitive strategic alliances. In my rush to make my plane, I neglected to specify in my meeting notes that a certain piece of information he'd shared was confidential. In a discussion with another strategic ally at the airport from a pay phone, I unwittingly betrayed that confidence. By the time I got off the plane in Florida, my boss was paging me on the loudspeakers at the airport. All hell had broken loose. The worst-case scenario was about to happen. The person whose confidence I'd betrayed had threatened to back out of the alliance. That meant that $70 million (!) was going down the drain—all because of me.

"My knees started to shake and I began to sweat as the entire nightmare grew worse and worse. Finally I got to my hotel and checked in. After reviewing the situation, I realized I had no alternative. I would just resign.

"Then I remembered Dr. Sha's healer-training program that I'd been taking to develop more creative abilities. A lot of the training dealt with the power of the mind and soul communication. Prayer was very important and necessary for self-healing and healing others. In essence, it was a way to alter the energy of a situation. So I walked outside the hotel (mainly because I was too nervous to stay inside) and began to call to the souls of all parties involved to reconnect and make peace.

"After just five minutes, a miracle happened. The bellhop came out and called for any person by my name to please come to the hotel phone. My heart raced as I dashed to the lobby.

"'Hello,' I said, my heart in my throat. It was my boss wanting me to know everything had been resolved and everyone was fine and still very supportive of the project. He wanted to call me so that I would not worry all weekend and be distracted giving the lecture.

"What a relief! I will never forget that I had the power to impact the situation in ways I never before understood. I hope I never have to use this process again. But it is great to know if you get yourself in a bad pinch."

As Andrew discovered, influencing the *chi* that surrounds you can greatly enhance your well-being on many different levels. If that doesn't work, however, you must look at what's going on inside you. So let's get back to the issue at hand, which is your health.

Just as with the furniture in your home, you want to promote the flow of *chi* in your body by removing any energy blockages and balancing the transformation between matter inside your cells and energy outside your cells. This will not only help you recover from unhealthy physical, mental, emotional, and spiritual conditions; it will give you power.

It all starts with the position of your hands in relation to your body and with the position of the body itself. Once you try this simple technique, you'll be amazed at how effective it can be.

"I use hands power especially when the transfer of energy is required to ease pain quickly and also to show the client the results and benefits of this kind of energy transfer," says Edwin Hood, a healer who studied with me in Canada. "By using the One Hand Near, One Hand Far Method, within a few minutes we can relieve headaches, toothaches, and most any kind of ache. For example, one hand is held near the high-energy field (e.g., the head, if one has a headache), while the other hand is held farther away facing the lower-energy field (e.g., the lower abdomen). Energy in the high-energy field is quickly transferred to the lower-energy area. I use this technique for balancing the client's energy and for reducing inflammation, pain, or discomfort. Because it works so effectively, I automatically use hands power at almost every healing session and on myself whenever I feel pain."

By creating fields of different intensities in relation to the body, hand positions can be used to transfer energy in the body for balancing and healing purposes. Let's say you have a headache. Whether you're suffering from a migraine or a dull pressure that simply won't go away, too much energy has accumulated in the area of your head. You can eliminate that with the One Hand Near, One Hand Far Method that Edwin just mentioned.

Healing Practice:
One Hand Near, One Hand Far
Hand Position

Place one hand 4 to 8 inches from the high-energy area (in the case of a headache, your head). That's called your near hand. Place your other hand (your far hand) 10 to 20 inches in front of your lower abdomen (or other area of your body that can use energy; the lower abdomen is good because it contains the Lower Dan Tian, an important energy center explained in depth in Chapter 11). The palms of both your hands should face your body.

Your near hand creates a high-density energy field, while your far hand creates a low-density energy field. Physics tells us that the energy in a high-density field flows to a low-density field naturally. It makes sense if you think about it. When you open a window in the wintertime, the cold and the wind flow in because of the high-density cold outside. So when you put one hand near and one hand far, you create a density difference, causing the energy that has accumulated in your head to flow naturally to your lower abdomen. If you want the result more quickly, you lower your far hand (the one by your belly) by 2 or 3 inches, and the excess energy will flow down even faster. Once that accumulation of energy has been dispersed, your headache will disappear.

You can also use this basic technique to relieve everything from inflammations, pain, and stiffness—all caused by an accumulation of excess energy—to stress and colds simply by placing the palm of the near hand facing toward the area being treated and the palm of the far hand toward an area in your body that can use more energy.

"On Wednesday my throat became so sore I could hardly swallow," says Pat. "My first line of defense, gargling and megadoses of echinacea, wasn't working as quickly as usual. So I decided to try the One Hand Near, One Hand Far Method for a sore throat. With my near hand 4 to 8 inches from my throat, and my far hand 10 to 20 inches away from my lower abdomen, I chanted the sounds of the numbers 1 and 9 ('ee-joe, ee-joe') and visualized a bright while light flowing from my throat to my lower abdomen. 'I love the soul of my throat,' I said out loud. 'Please help to promote *chi* flow and blood flow. Be light and transparent. Get well. Thank you, thank, you, thank you.' Each time I did the exercise, my throat pain would go away. After practicing the exercise three or four times, my sore throat was gone!

"Next came the runny nose on Thursday. My husband had just spent several nights awake with a box of tissues. I certainly didn't relish the prospect of going through the same experience. I did Dr. Sha's hand self-healing for a runny nose several times that evening. With the palm of my near hand facing my chest, held 4 to 8 inches out and just above the level of my nipples, and my far hand held 10 to 20 inches out facing the side of my body at chest level, I chanted the natural sounds of the numbers 3 and 5 ('sahn-woo, sahn-woo'), visualized a white light flowing from my nose down to my stomach, and asked the soul of my lungs and the soul of my nose to please vibrate and promote the flow of *chi* in those areas. Then I thanked them three times as always, and slept through the night. When I awoke on Friday, I had no sign of the bad head cold." You probably noticed that Pat, in addition to the One Hand Near, One Hand Far Method, also used three other power self-healing techniques. Although those may sound funny to you right now, they'll make total sense when I explain them later on in the book. This will help you the next time you need to clear up coldlike symptoms, so it bears repeating step by step.

You can clear up a stuffed or runny nose simply by placing your near hand 4 to 8 inches away from the middle of your chest, above the level of your nipples, and your far hand 10 to 20 inches from the side of your body at chest level. In a strong voice, chant the words *san wu* (Chinese for the numbers 3 and 5, pronounced "sahn-woo") so that the sound vibrations help dispel the blocked energy in your lungs that has caused your nose to become congested. Then visualize a light flowing from your nose down to your stomach. Finally, even though it probably sounds strange right now, ask for help from the souls of your lungs and your nose, just like Pat did. Do all this for five minutes, and repeat the procedure several times during a day.

But I'm getting ahead of myself.

Three other very important body power techniques will serve you well in the months and years to come. The Open *San Jiao* Body Power Technique is fundamental for self-healing any physical problem because it promotes *chi* flow and blood flow throughout the *San Jiao*, which includes most of the body and all the major organs. The *Yin/Yang* Palm Body Power Technique builds up the foundation power of the body. This is critical for increasing immunity, preventing illness, and prolonging life. The *Xiu Lian* Body Power Technique to increase intelligence helps develop the potential power of the brain. It can also be used to help unlock the spiritual capabilities of the Third Eye and the Message Center.

These body power techniques will bring great blessings for your healing journey, and for your spiritual journey as well. Practice them, enjoy them, and gain the benefits.

OPEN *SAN JIAO* BODY POWER TECHNIQUE

In traditional Chinese medicine, *San Jiao* (pronounced "sahn jow") is the name for the three major areas in our body. *San* means "three." *Jiao* means "area." The three areas—the Upper, Middle, and Lower *Jiao*—include the major organs and the space around the organs.

The Upper *Jiao* is defined as the area between the top of the head and the diaphragm. This area includes the brain, heart, lungs, bronchial tubes, and the space around these organs. Put your hand on your chest. This is the Upper *Jiao* area. The main function of the Upper *Jiao* is to promote *chi* and blood circulation in the whole body.

The Middle *Jiao* is defined as the area from the diaphragm to the level of the navel. Put your hand just above your navel. This is the Middle *Jiao* area. The Middle *Jiao* includes the spleen, stomach, liver, pancreas, and the space around these organs. The main function of the Middle *Jiao* is the transportation and transformation of food and water. The Middle *Jiao* also absorbs nutrients to support the production of blood.

The Lower *Jiao* is defined as the area from the level of the navel to the level of the genitals. Put your hand just below your navel. This is the Lower *Jiao* area. The kidneys, small intestine, large intestine, urinary bladder, female organs such as the uterus and ovaries, male organs such as the testicles and prostate, and the space around these organs are in the Lower *Jiao*. One of the main functions of the Lower *Jiao* is to produce energy. The other main functions of the Lower *Jiao* are the elimination of bodily waste and superfluous water and the control of the reproductive system.

San Jiao is the pathway of *chi* in the whole body. *San Jiao* is also the pathway of water in the whole body. For good health, *chi* and bodily fluids must flow smoothly in the *San Jiao*.

Healing Practice
Body Position

For the basic standing position, totally relax your body. Place your feet shoulder-width apart. Bend your knees slightly. Contract your anus slightly.[1] Keep your back straight. Touch the tip of your tongue to the roof of your mouth and maintain this contact to promote the flow of *chi*.

Hand Position

Place your right hand 3 inches above the navel, with palm facing up. If you have hypertension, a headache, a brain tumor, or cancer, then place your right palm facing down. Place your left hand 3 inches below the navel, with palm facing up. Smile slightly. (See Figure 1.)

Practice Time

If you are healthy, practice fifteen minutes at a time in the basic standing position for the prevention of sickness. For energy boosting and self-healing, practice at least thirty minutes to create and promote energy flow in the *San Jiao* areas. For cancer and other life-threatening conditions and to build strong immunity

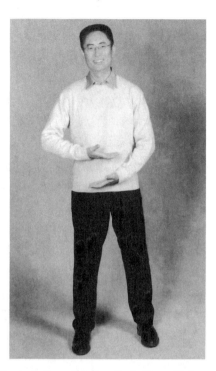

Figure 1. Open San Jiao Body Power Technique

and great self-healing power, you must practice at least one hour at a time, the longer the better.

If you are very sick and weak, start by practicing only five minutes at a time. Increase the time gradually as you gain strength, attempting to work up to one hour or more. In China, many people with chronic and life-threatening conditions practice this particular technique for two hours or more at a time, aware of the self-healing that the Open *San Jiao* Body Power Technique has been proven to promote. If you are too weak to stand, please sit or lie down to begin this practice. After you feel better, start to practice in a standing position, even for a short period of time.

Why does the Open *San Jiao* Body Power Technique work? In this position, the right hand is placed just above the navel, which stimulates the Middle *Jiao*. Major organs such as the spleen, stomach, liver, gall bladder, and pancreas are located in the Middle *Jiao*. The right hand radiates energy to stimulate the major organs in the Middle *Jiao*, causing these organs to radiate more energy themselves. This energy will stimulate the Upper *Jiao*, which includes major organs such as the brain, heart, lungs, and bronchial tubes. It is a chain reaction. The organs in the Upper *Jiao* will vibrate more, causing energy to radiate up to the brain, stimulating more vibration in the brain cells. This chain reaction explains why placing the right hand in front of the Middle *Jiao* will promote energy flow all the way from the Middle *Jiao* to the top of the head.

Now, let me explain what the left hand is doing. In this position, the left hand is placed in front of the Lower *Jiao*. Major organs such as the kidneys, small intestine, large intestine, urinary bladder, female organs (uterus and ovaries) and male organs (prostate and testicles) are located in the Lower *Jiao*. The left hand radiates energy to stimulate the vibration of these organs in the Lower *Jiao*. These organs will then radiate more energy to stimulate the vibration of the legs at the thigh level. The vibration of the thighs will then stimulate the vibration of the knees. In this chain reaction, the vibration will increase all the way from the Lower *Jiao* to the toes.

As you now know, by using the Open *San Jiao* Body Power Technique, your right hand will promote energy flow from the Middle *Jiao* up to the head, and your left hand will promote energy flow from the Lower *Jiao* to your toes. This body power technique will therefore promote energy flow in your whole body. As explained earlier, every sickness is caused by imbalance in the flow of *chi*. Promoting the flow of *chi* will help every unhealthy condition recover.

Please understand that a person with chronic pain or illness or life-threatening conditions such as cancer has a serious energy blockage. It takes time to remove an energy blockage. I repeat, for self-healing, the Open *San Jiao* Body Power Technique must be practiced at least thirty minutes at a time. A person with a life-threatening condition must practice at least one hour at a time, as many times a day as possible.

Remember that it takes time to recover from your unhealthy conditions. Always remind yourself of these few key words when you practice this or any other self-healing technique in this book:

Patience

Confidence

Practice hard

Self-healing benefits will bless you

When you practice the Open *San Jiao* Body Power Technique for a while, you will feel warm and energetic and experience a tingling sensation in your body. You will feel that you are healing your body, mind, and soul.

Increase the time you practice with every session. You will definitely feel the energy when you are able to stand for a half hour per session. When you can stand for one hour per session, you will definitely feel increased inner healing power and strength. This technique is very simple, but very practical and powerful. You will receive great benefits to heal body, mind, and soul by practicing it seriously, happily, and willingly. The Open *San Jiao* Body Power Technique will promote energy flow to every part of the body. It will remove the energy blockages. Healing blessings are waiting for you, so start practicing!

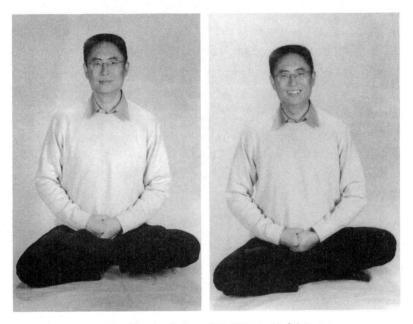

Figure 2. Full Lotus (left) and Half Lotus (right) Positions

YIN/YANG PALM BODY POWER TECHNIQUE

The *Yin/Yang* Palm Body Power Technique will help you develop power in the Lower *Dan Tian* (pronounced "dahn tee-en") and Snow Mountain Area, two of the most important energy centers in the body (which I'll discuss in detail later). Increasing the power in these two energy centers is the key to increasing immunity and stamina and prolonging life.

Healing Practice
Body Position

The best body position is to sit in a full lotus. If you are unable to sit in a full lotus, you may adopt a half lotus position or simply cross your legs naturally. (See Figure 2.) Sitting on a chair is also fine, but be sure to keep your feet flat on the floor. You can even

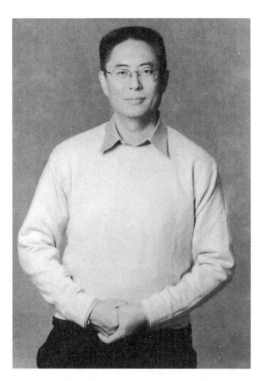

Figure 3. Yin/Yang Palm Body Power Technique

practice this body power technique lying in bed The important thing in any position is to keep your whole body relaxed.

Hand Position

With the fingers of your right hand, grasp your left thumb tightly and make a fist. Your right hand should grasp your left thumb with 70–80 percent of your maximum strength. Let the fingers of your left hand rest naturally on the top of your right hand. You have now transformed your palms into the *Yin/Yang* palm. (See Figure 3.) Keeping your grip on your left thumb, place your *Yin/Yang* palm on your lower abdomen, just below your navel.

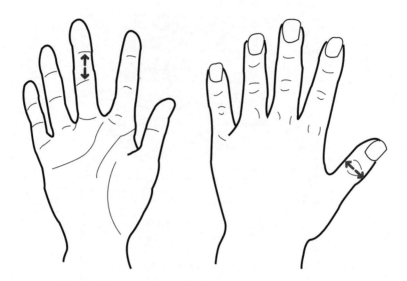

Figure 4. Personal Body Inch Measurement (Cun)

Practice Time

Continue to hold the *Yin/Yang* palm on your lower abdomen for at least fifteen minutes, the longer the better.

There are two important energy centers inside your lower abdomen. The Lower *Dan Tian* is a fist-sized energy center found 1½ *cun* below the navel and 2½ *cun* inside the body. The *cun* (pronounced "tsuen") is defined as the width of the top joint of the thumb at its widest point. Alternatively, it is the distance from the top crease to the middle crease (not the joint length) of the middle finger, on the palm side of the finger. (See Figure 4.) The Snow Mountain Area is found by drawing an imaginary line straight through from the navel to the small of the back. From the back point, go in one-third of this line and down 2½ *cun* (just in front of your spinal column). The *Yin/Yang* Palm Body Power Technique stimulates these two energy centers in the lower abdomen, promoting cellular vibration in the entire lower abdomen.

The hand position of the *Yin/Yang* Palm Body Power Technique requires that the right palm grasp the left thumb tightly. The thumb represents the energy of the spleen and stomach. For five thousand years of Chinese history, energy specialists and spiritual practitioners have understood that each finger is associated with certain major organs. This association is an energy connection. According to Zhi Neng medicine, the thumb represents spleen and stomach, the index finger represents liver and gall bladder, the middle finger represents heart and small intestine, the ring finger represents lungs and large intestine, and the little finger represents kidneys and urinary bladder.

When you squeeze your left thumb in the *Yin/Yang* Palm Body Power Technique, you will accelerate the cellular vibration of your spleen and stomach. This vibration will improve the functioning of your digestive system. You will digest food and absorb nutrients well.

XIU LIAN BODY POWER TECHNIQUE

For five thousand years, *Xiu Lian* (pronounced "shoo lee-en") has been one of the most important practices in Chinese spiritual study. *Xiu* means to purify your heart, mind, and soul. It means having love, care, compassion, sincerity, honesty, generosity, integrity, unselfishness, and discipline. It also means accumulating virtue and giving service to people and society. *Lian* means to practice all of these things in your daily life, in your actions, behaviors, and thoughts.

Buddhists, Taoists, Confucians, and energy and spiritual practitioners all know the term *Xiu Lian*, which carries a great variety and richness of meaning. To do a good job in *Xiu Lian* may take an entire lifetime because it requires discipline and service. It also takes a person a lifetime of practicing *Xiu Lian* to improve his or her life. It requires contributing one's heart and capabilities to people and to society. It requires enlightening one's heart and one's soul with service. For success with *Xiu Lian*, every person should know it takes a lot of hard work to do better and better.

For *Xiu Lian*, beneficial thoughts must constantly be translated into action. That is why *Xiu Lian* is such a popular concept in energy and spiritual study and in Buddhism, Taoism, and Confucianism. *Xiu Lian* has also been used for the entire five-thousand-year history of Chinese culture to describe a person's individual spiritual journey, especially the soul's journey.

Why do people practice *Xiu Lian*? The first purpose of *Xiu Lian* is enlightenment of the soul. People who practice *Xiu Lian* seriously want their souls to be pure and they want to acquire soul capabilities. The main purpose of *Xiu Lian* is to be aware of soul issues and prepare your soul so that it goes to the best place when your physical life ends.

The second purpose of *Xiu Lian* is to develop the intelligence of your mind and soul. People who practice *Xiu Lian* want to develop their brain capabilities and soul capabilities in order to serve people, society, and the world. Your record of service to people, society, and the world is called virtue, or *te* (pronounced "duh," a Taoist term), in ancient Chinese philosophy. The Buddhist name for this record of service or virtue is *karma*. People who do *Xiu Lian* gain good *te*, good karma, good virtue. Why do they do this? They want their souls to go to the best place after their physical bodies die. The third purpose of *Xiu Lian* is to strengthen the body's energy and to be healthier and happier in one's physical life.

A person who practices *Xiu Lian* must recognize that this practice has two main goals for the physical body. One goal is to build up foundation power to strengthen the immune system, improve the quality of life, and prolong life. The other goal for the body in *Xiu Lian* practice is to develop the intelligence of the mind and the soul. The key energy centers to develop the intelligence of the mind and soul are the Message Center and Third Eye. Developing the Message Center gives you the capability to converse directly with God, your Heaven Team, and any soul in the universe. Opening the Third Eye gives you the capability to see the image of God, your Heaven Team, and any soul in the universe.

The *Xiu Lian* Body Power Technique has proven to be a powerful way to develop the intelligence of the mind and the soul. It develops the Message Center to talk directly with the soul world and helps open the Third Eye to see the soul world. The Message Center of the body is the Middle *Dan Tian*. It is one of the five key energy centers of the body, which I'll discuss in greater detail later on. It is a fist-sized area starting from the point midway between the nipples. The Third Eye is the Upper *Dan Tian*. It is also one of the five key energy centers of the body. It is a cherry-sized area located near the center of the head, in the area of the pineal gland.

Healing Practice
Body Position

Sit comfortably with your back straight, but not leaning against anything. Keep both feet on the floor. Relax.

Hand Position

Place your hands in front of your chest. Gently touch the heels of your hands together, gently touch your thumbs together, and

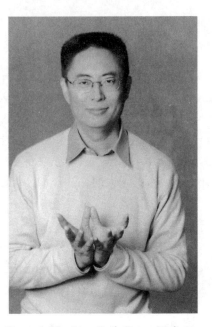

Figure 5. Xiu Lian Body Power Technique

gently touch your little fingers together. Open your hands and fingers as though you were holding a beautiful lotus flower. (See Figure 5.)

Practice Time

Relax and maintain the position for a few minutes—the longer the better—while your mind is in a peaceful, pleasant, or meditative state.

Those weren't too hard were they? And just wait and see what they can do for you! Still, as powerful as the body power techniques you've just learned are by themselves, they are all that and more when combined with the three other power-healing techniques I'm about to share with you. So let's move on to sound power.

8

SOUND POWER

Try this. Put your hands out in front of you and extend your two index fingers so they're parallel to one another. Keeping your fingers and hands relaxed, close your eyes and repeat the following phrase: "Fingers come together, fingers come together, fingers come together." Within three minutes, without any conscious effort on your part, your fingers will have done just that: they will have come together. You can try the same thing with your hands ("Hands come together") or arms ("Arms come together"), and it will work exactly the same way.

Why? Because that's the power of sound. Just as you can create a direction for your energy to flow through your intense desire to get well and by using body power techniques, you can achieve remarkable results through the voiced power of suggestion and sound power techniques. Actually, "suggestion" isn't quite the right word, because instead of suggesting that your body can heal itself, you're going to be commanding your body to do just that.

Sound also serves to vibrate your organs, thereby stimulating and accelerating the flow of energy. Chant the mantra *"Weng ar hong"* (pronounced "wung ar hohng") and you'll see—and feel—

what I mean for yourself. Before chanting each sound take a deep breath so that, just like carrying a note when you sing, you allow each sound to resonate as long as possible. "Wuuuunnnnngggggggg, aaaaaarrrrrrrr, hoooohnnnngggg." As you chant the first sound, *weng*, place your hand on your cheek, then on your neck. You'll feel both areas vibrating. If you touch your chest while chanting the next sound, *ar*, you'll feel the vibration there. With the last sound, *hong*, you can feel your belly vibrate.

Healing happens when you combine these vibrations with the special message inherent in a mantra. In fact, that's exactly what mantras are: special sounds created by God, spiritual leaders, or other enlightened persons that are effective whether they are said aloud or silently. Mantras are very powerful and have already benefited millions of people by healing their bodies, minds, and souls and by blessing their work, relationships, and life journeys. This explains why more and more people throughout the world are using mantras for healing and blessing.

In India, mantras are chanted for hours, days, or years according to the instructions given to the student by the teacher. Ordinary homemakers use mantras as prayers to signal the passage of time in the day, saying an opening mantra at daybreak, another at noon, and still another at sunset. Muslims say prayers throughout the day and night, giving out the message of Allah. Hindu believers sing *bhajans* for hours, sometimes day and night, when an ashram is celebrating an important holy day. In the West, sound is woven into many religious services. In Christian countries, hymns, gospels, songs, and other forms of music are standard in religious services.

Although people around the world use sound differently, when it comes to healing, it's all about communicating and asking for what you want. You must tell the body how to do the work in no uncertain terms. This is not the time for tentative, little voices.

You must sound loud, dynamic (even emphatic), and supremely confident.

Research has shown that attitude influences our state of health and our potential for recovery. I remember a man with an itchy foot fungus that was driving him mad. Nothing he had tried had gotten rid of the irritation that was tormenting him. Finally he broke down and started to yell at the foot fungus, no less. "Go away! I hate you," he screamed. "I don't want to live with you anymore. Go away and leave me alone!" You know what? His foot fungus disappeared. His will, which he had finally communicated in no uncertain terms, commanded his body to get rid of the fungus—and it did.

Love can be even more powerful when communicated to various parts of your body. How did Paul manage to self-heal himself right out of the emergency room after suffering an asthma attack that normally would have hospitalized him or worse? "I learned to talk to my lungs and to love them, not hate them," he says. "I began to talk to my lungs every day on the way to work as I chanted the mantras on the tape. I felt hopeful. I began to practice the energy-developing techniques, and I became more energized. Shortly after returning from the hospital I developed a fever from a secondary bacterial infection. I am glad to report that my lungs stayed clear. I can attest that prior to implementing Dr. Sha's self-healing techniques my lungs never reversed themselves once an attack had started. Personally, I plan to make a life study out of energy healing and the art of talking to my body, mind, and soul."

For over five thousand years, Buddhists, Taoists and Confucians (the three main spiritual groups in Chinese cultural history) have applied sound power techniques for healing and blessing. They've also been used by many others in China, including traditional Chinese medicine and qigong practitioners.

Why have many people throughout the East used mantras through the ages to bless their work, relationships, and lives? Because a mantra is a message, very much like a prayer. When you chant a mantra over and over, you send a request to the mantra. Mantra is the spirit. Mantra is the message. Mantra is the soul. You get a blessing from this special spirit, message, or soul. People who receive a blessing from a mantra do not always understand why. This blessing comes because a special spirit, message, or soul is blessing you.

A mantra is a special message created by God or by a special person. The mantra is used to communicate and commune with literally millions of people to share love, care, compassion, sincerity, honesty, and generosity and to support and heal one another. When you practice a special mantra, it is as though you are telephoning or e-mailing millions of people who practice the same mantra.

At the message level, every one of these fellow mantra practitioners knows that you need help at that very moment. They send back good messages to you to help you in whatever you request. This is why the mantra is so powerful. The thoughts and souls of millions of people are helping you. At the same moment, millions of people are healing your body, mind, and soul and blessing your other requests. This brings incredible results to your health and to your life's journey. This is how miracles occur.

"Early this year, I experienced a disconcerting heartbeat irregularity associated with a chronic allergic condition," recalls Harry. "Neither my internist nor my cardiologist could successfully bring it under control, although they continued to monitor it closely over the course of a few months. I turned to Dr. Sha, who developed a healing protocol and assisted me in administering it over the telephone. My main self-healing practice was simply to chant the natural sound of the number 2 (in Chinese *'Ar, ar, ar, ar . . . '*) to stimulate cellular vibration in and around my heart. After five days, my heart palpitations disappeared, and the severity of the allergic reaction was curtailed substantially. Nothing else had worked."

Today millions of people around the world use this ancient technique to heal body, mind, and soul.

Remember Pat, who was able to alleviate her sore throat and runny nose using the One Hand Near, One Hand Far Method? Just a few days later, while on a trip that couldn't be postponed, she realized that the virus she had been battling had settled into her lungs. Of course, having been out in the rain, wind, and cold during her travels hadn't helped her condition. Her chest quickly became congested, and she began coughing huskily. Having a history of bronchitis and pneumonia, she knew the feeling all too well. But many "sahn-sahn's" (the natural sound of the number 3 to vibrate the chest and lungs) later, along with a drink of hot ginger, lemon, garlic, and honey, her coughing stopped. Once again, she slept through the night and was completely clear a day and a half later. "No antibiotics, just some remedies from nature and Dr. Sha's power-healing techniques," she says. "Thank you, Dr. Sha!"

Then there's Peggy, a single mother who recently started her own business. Though she was excited about the new venture, she was feeling somewhat stressed at having to handle all the aspects of her new business while still caring for her two children. As she was preparing for a very important business meeting, she noticed she had a stomachache. She knew she had to attend this meeting no matter how she felt, so she tried ignoring her stomachache. As she started her commute, the pains became really awful. She knew she would be in the car for the next thirty minutes with no access to any medication. She felt trapped, but had to continue to her meeting. She started using the self-healing techniques by repeating over and over: "woo-joe" (the number 5, *wu,* pronounced "woo," for the stomach, and the number 9, *jiu,* pronounced "joe," for the lower abdomen) and "Light flows down." It was her intention to send the excess energy in her stomach, which she thought was the cause of her pain, down to her lower abdomen. She repeated "woo-joe" and "Light flows down" over and over and over during her thirty-minute commute. When she arrived at her meeting, her stomachache was gone and she felt very relaxed. Not surprisingly, her meeting went very well.

Each mantra has its own message. Some mantras have a special message for healing or for developing energy. Some mantras have a special message for opening your Third Eye or your Message Center to converse directly with God and your Heaven Team. Others have a special message for blessing or protecting your life. A powerful mantra may include many special messages.

Every mantra also has a special sound. That sound vibrates different parts of the body. That sound carries special energy. That sound can be used for healing, blessing, protecting, and improving the quality of your cells, organs, and body.

When you practice a mantra, you do not say it only once. You do not say it only a few times. When you chant a mantra, you should practice a half hour, an hour, even many hours. Why? Suppose that you chant a mantra to remove your energy blockage at the cellular level. The power of the mantra can do this. The special message and the special sound of the mantra will stimulate the vibration of the cells and organs. The mantra will balance the transformation between the matter inside the cells and the energy outside the cells. This balance takes time to be accomplished. That is why one of the common characteristics of mantra use is repetitive practice, saying the mantra over and over and over and over.

Let's go back to our headache example to see how effective mantras can be. As I'm sure you remember, headaches are caused by too much energy accumulated in the head area. We discussed how by placing one hand near and one hand far, you can cause that energy to relocate to the lower abdomen. Sounds will also help transfer this excess energy, speeding it along its way, thereby accelerating the relief you feel.

Of course, this doesn't just work on headaches. Linda, a secretary whose severe tendonitis jeopardized her job and left her incapable of even driving a car, relieved that excruciating condition with a mantra. Along the way, her persistent constipation and bleeding hemorrhoids also cleared up.

"I am an administrator in a software company," she writes. "My responsibilities involve a lot of computer work and keeping things organized for the executives. About four years ago, I had very severe pain in my right arm, to the point where I could barely use it at times and couldn't lift it. None of my doctors could find anything wrong. All they could tell me was that I probably had tendonitis and might have to keep my arm in a cast to rest it.

"After a few months, the pain subsided for a while simply because I started learning how to use and rely more on my left arm, while using my right arm less. But then in May 2000 I was in a car accident, and the pain returned. I started seeing an acupuncturist every week who used traditional acupuncture as well as electro-acupuncture. But even with all these treatments, my progress was up and down. Sometimes I felt better, but at other times the pain would be back again. Overall, there really wasn't much change over the five or six months I got these treatments.

"In addition, I started to suffer from back pain. I had no idea what caused it, and my doctors couldn't tell me either. I thought it might be a problem with my liver or my kidneys, so I had those tested, but they were okay. My doctor said, 'You probably just pulled a muscle.' My response was, 'How could I have pulled a muscle? All I did was rest at home for a few days. Then when I went to work, I couldn't sit, I couldn't walk.'

"That's when someone in my office said, 'Why don't you see Dr. Sha?' Incredibly, after just a couple of sessions with Dr. Sha, I was all better! More important, he also taught me how to help myself. I have a long, slow commute to work and drive a stick shift. All the shifting sometimes causes my pains to act up. I chant on my way to work and back, trying to visualize light—while keeping my eyes on the road of course! After a few minutes, I realize that my pains have gone away! I also chant "God's light" and visualize the light in my back and, somehow, the pain just disappears. That's when I realize that this stuff really works!

"I've also suffered from a very bad, chronic case of constipation, to the extent where I would bleed at times. And my doctors would tell me, 'Oh, you have a bad case of hemorrhoids. You can come in and have them cut out.' That was the only solution they could give me. But when I started chanting the number 9 (*jiu,* "joe"), the constipation problem went away within a month. It really works! I may still have hemorrhoids, but they've shrunk, and I definitely don't have any more problems going to the bathroom."

When you practice mantras, there are two ways to chant: aloud or silently. Chanting the sound aloud vibrates the bigger cells in your body. Chanting silently vibrates the smaller cells in your body. Both ways are important, and you need to practice both.

To use mantras, you'll want to:

- Sit or lie down comfortably.

- Calm your mind and heart.

- Show respect for the mantra.

- Totally relax.
- Call the mantra a few times.
- Tell the mantra what you need for healing and blessing.
- Say "Thank you, thank you, thank you" to show gratitude and honor. The first "thank you" is to God, the second, to the members of your Heaven Team, and the third, to your own body, mind, and soul.
- Start to chant. You may chant any mantra aloud or silently and still gain the benefits.
- Visualize light if so indicated in a given exercise. This is a mind power technique.
- As you begin to chant, don't think about anything. Just chant the mantra and visualize light.
- Chant as long as you can. Again, you may chant aloud or silently.
- When you are finished, say again "Thank you, thank you, thank you."
- Send the message of the mantra back to the spiritual world by saying, "The spirit of the mantra, and all the other spirits who are here, could you please return to the spiritual world?"

Why send the mantra back? At the beginning of the mantra practice, you requested a mantra, which is a spirit, a soul, or a message, to come join you. During the practice, the spirit has been with you. After ending the practice, say "Thank you" and respectfully return the spirit to the spiritual world. This is a soul power technique.

Applying these important procedures properly—without skipping a single step—is vital for self-healing, for healing others, and for blessing your work, family, and entire life. Do them right, and you'll be amazed at how far-reaching and life-altering their impact can be.

Over the course of Chinese history, millions of people have experienced the benefits of using the following mantras.

WENG AR HONG

The powerful mantra *Weng ar hong* (pronounced "wung ar hohng"), used by millions of spiritual practitioners throughout China and other countries to heal unhealthy conditions throughout the body, vibrates the *San Jiao* (which includes all the major organs) to promote *chi* flow for self-healing. As you already know from our recent experiment, *weng* vibrates the entire head, *ar* vibrates the whole chest, and *hong* vibrates the whole abdomen.

When you chant this mantra, which can also be used as a blessing for your business, relationships, and success, visualize different colored lights in the Upper, Middle, and Lower *Jiao* of your body. There are two ways to visualize the lights during your practice:

- To emphasize developing the wisdom and capabilities of the brain and opening the Third Eye, visualize bright white light radiating in your head as you chant *"weng."* When you chant *"ar,"* visualize bright red light radiating in your chest. When you chant *"hong,"* visualize bright blue light radiating in your abdomen. This mind power technique is used by Tibetan spiritual practitioners.

- To emphasize healing for the body, mind, and soul, visualize bright red light radiating in your head as you chant *"weng."* When you chant *"ar,"* visualize bright white light radiating in your chest. When you chant *"hong,"* visualize bright blue light radiating in your abdomen. This mind power technique is used by Zhi Neng medicine practitioners.

You can practice either or both techniques depending on your emphasis.

Healing Practice
Body Position (Body Power Technique)

Stand with your feet shoulder-width apart. Keep your knees slightly bent. Contract your anus slightly. Keep your back straight.

Hand Position (Body Power Technique)

Put one hand 4 to 8 inches above your head, palm facing down. Put your other hand 12 to 20 inches above your head, palm facing down.

Communicate (Soul Power Technique)

"*Weng ar hong, weng ar hong, weng ar hong, weng ar hong,* could you help me solve my problem [name whatever physical, emotional, mental, or spiritual problem you are requesting help for]? Thank you, thank you, thank you."

Chant (Sound Power Technique)

Inhale deeply. As you exhale slowly, chant *"Weng ar hong"* in one breath. Repeat as many times as you can.

Visualize (Mind Power Technique)

As you chant, visualize light radiating in different parts of your body. Follow the different color instructions in one of the two techniques explained on page 90. As you repeat the mantra, visualize the colored lights getting brighter and brighter.

Close (Soul Power Technique)

Say "*Hao, hao, hao* (*hao,* pronounced 'how,' means 'Get well,' 'Get stronger'). Thank you, thank you, thank you."

Practice Time

Repeat this mantra as long as you can per session, as many times a day as you can.

Blessing Practice

For blessing your business, your relationships, and your life, you can vary the above practice.

In place of the request for help with a problem, say "*Weng ar hong, weng ar hong, weng ar hong, weng ar hong.* Could you bless me [make your request for blessing]?" Proceed as above by taking a deep breath and, as you exhale slowly, chanting *"Weng ar hong"* in one breath. At the same time, visualize different colors of light radiating in different parts of the body, using one of the two techniques explained on page 90. Visualize the colored lights becoming brighter and brighter.

AR MI TUO FUO

Ar Mi Tuo Fuo (pronounced "ar mee toe foe") is one of the most popular and powerful Buddhist mantras in history. Buddhists believe there is a spiritual world in heaven named *Ji Le Shi Jie*, the World of Most Happiness. (*Ji* means "most." *Le* means "happiness." *Shi Jie* means "world.") There are countless Buddhas in that spiritual world and Ar Mi Tuo Fuo is their leader. Millions of Buddhists apply this mantra for healing and blessing and for spiritual enlightenment.

This mantra is very powerful for fully opening the Message Center to converse directly with the soul world. It is also powerful for purifying your body, mind, and soul and for attaining peace.

Healing Practice
Body Position (Body Power Technique)

Sit in a full or half lotus position (see Figure 2 in Chapter 7) or naturally cross your legs. You may sit in a chair, but do not cross your ankles or legs and keep your feet flat on the floor. Keep your back away from (not touching) the backrest. Relax your whole body.

Hand Position (Body Power Technique)

Place your hands in the prayer position in front of your chest, palms as close as possible but not touching. (See Figure 6.)

Communicate (Soul Power Technique)

Say "*Ar Mi Tuo Fuo, Ar Mi Tuo Fuo, Ar Mi Tuo Fuo, Ar Mi Tuo Fuo*, could you help me [make your request for health, for blessing, for your business or relationships, for opening your Message Center, or for purifying your soul or your heart]?" Say "Thank you, thank you, thank you" to express gratitude to the mantra.

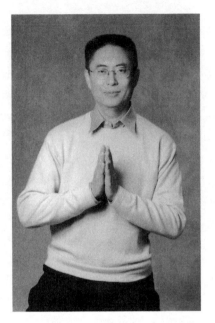

Figure 6. Prayer Hands Body Power Technique

Chant (Sound Power Technique)

Chant "*Ar Mi Tuo Fuo, Ar Mi Tuo Fuo, Ar Mi Tuo Fuo, Ar Mi Tuo Fuo*" continuously.

Close (Soul Power Technique)

Say "*Hao, hao, hao.* Thank you, thank you, thank you."

Practice Time

Repeat the mantra for as long as you can per session, as many times a day as you can.

Let me emphasize again, healing your unhealthy conditions and blessing your life both take time. Be patient and confident. Trust the power of the mantra. Healing and blessing will come to you.

Weng Ma Ni Ba Ma Hong

Weng ma ni ba ma hong (pronounced "wung mah nee bah mah hohng") is the mantra of Guan Shi Yin, one of the most famous Buddhas. This Buddha is known as the Compassion Buddha. *Guan* means "see" and "hear." *Shi* means "world." *Yin* means "condition" and "voice." The Compassion Buddha sees the world's condition and hears the world's voice, with great compassion. Millions of people in the history of China, including millions of Buddhists, have practiced this mantra. This mantra has great healing and blessing power. During the 1950s, a famous Buddhist monk shared the body power technique for applying this great mantra.

Healing Practice
Body Position (Body Power Technique)

Sit in a full or half lotus position (see Figure 2 in Chapter 7) or with naturally crossed legs. You may sit in a chair with your feet flat on the floor. Keep your back away from (not touching) the backrest.

Hand Position (Body Power Technique)

Place your hands in front of your chest. Gently touch the heels of your hands together, gently touch your thumbs together, and gently touch your little fingers together. Open your hands and fingers as though you were holding a beautiful lotus flower. (See Figure 5 in Chapter 7.)

Communicate (Soul Power Technique)

Say "*Weng ma ni ba ma hong, weng ma ni ba ma hong, weng ma ni ba ma hong, weng ma ni ba ma hong,* could you help me [make

your request for health, for blessings in work, for blessings in relationships, etc.]?" Say "Thank you, thank you, thank you" to
express gratitude to the mantra.

Chant (Sound Power Technique)

Chant *"Weng ma ni ba ma hong, weng ma ni ba ma hong, weng ma
ni ba ma hong, weng ma ni ba ma hong"* for as long as you can.

Visualize (Mind Power Technique)

While you are chanting, visualize bright white light in any part of
your body.

Close (Soul Power Technique)

Say *"Hao, hao, hao.* Thank you, thank you, thank you."

Practice Time

Repeat the mantra for as long as you can per session, as many
times a day as you can.

NATURAL NUMBER SOUNDS, 1–11

For more than five thousand years, Chinese medicine has used
special healing sounds to vibrate and heal the internal organs. For
example, traditional Chinese medicine has used *jiao* (pronounced
"jow") to vibrate the liver. *Zhi* (pronounced "djih") vibrates the
heart. *Gong* (pronounced "gohng") vibrates the spleen. *Shang*
(pronounced "shahng") vibrates the lungs. *Yu* (pronounced "yih")
vibrates the kidneys.

Buddhists and Taoists apply many mantras to vibrate specific parts of the body. For example, earlier in this chapter we introduced the mantra *Weng ar hong.* Recall that *weng* vibrates the Upper *Jiao*, *ar* vibrates the Middle *Jiao,* and *hong* vibrates the Lower *Jiao*.

As you felt for yourself, sound has a vibrational effect on various parts of the body. Indeed, sound *is* vibration. My teacher, Dr. Zhi Chen Guo, discovered in meditation practice that the natural sounds in Mandarin Chinese of the numbers from 1 through 11 vibrate different parts of the body. When he chanted these different number sounds, he could feel different parts of his body vibrating. Through his Third Eye, he could also see the vibration in the different parts of his body.

Since then, Master Guo has taught millions how to use these number sounds for healing and self-healing. Their experience shows that the healing effects are real.

The following example will show you how it works. The number 9, *jiu,* is pronounced "joe." This natural number sound vibrates the lower abdomen. Try this for yourself. Put one palm on your navel and chant "Joe, joe, joe, joe, joe, joe, joe, joe." Feel the vibration in your lower abdomen.

One of my clients, an attorney, suffered from constipation for more than ten years. Every day, she had to ingest fiber to have a bowel movement. I taught her to chant the natural sound of the number 9, "joe, joe, joe, joe," five minutes at a time, five times a day. After one week, she told me very excitedly that she no longer suffered from constipation. It is now four years later and she has been fine the whole time. In fact, I have had many clients who have successfully used the natural sound of the number 9 to solve their constipation problems.

Another client, an elderly woman, was hospitalized after suffering a heart attack. After recovering to the point where she was released from the hospital, she used the natural sound of the number 2, *ar* (pronounced "ar"), which vibrates the heart. My client chanted this sound a great deal every day, literally for hours: "Ar, ar, ar, ar, ar, ar, ar, ar." While she chanted, she visualized light radiating in her heart (a mind power technique). She talked with her heart (a soul power technique): "I love my heart. I love my heart." She also used the One Hand Near, One Hand Far Method that I've taught you. She practiced all the self-healing she'd learned with great discipline. After just two weeks, she reported what a difference they'd made. She said her heartbeat was very stable and circulation in her whole body was much better. Now, three years later, she is fine and continues this practice.

To sum up, Zhi Neng medicine uses the Mandarin pronunciation[1] of numbers and sounds to develop energy and to balance energy for health. Repeating different numbers causes different parts of the body to vibrate and resonate. These natural number sounds stimulate cellular vibration. Then, the flow of energy in the area increases, resulting in enhanced energy and better health.

These simple, practical, and powerful sounds are used throughout this book as part of many different self-healing techniques. Pay attention to them. These healing sounds will serve you very well, sometimes in ways that you can't possibly anticipate.

The numbers, their natural sounds, and the parts of the body they stimulate are shown in Table 1 on the next page.

Table 1
Natural Number Sounds, 1 to 11

Number	Mandarin Chinese	Pronunciation	Area Stimulated
1	*yi* or *yao*	ee or yow	head, brain
2	*ar*	ar	heart
3	*san*	sahn	chest, lungs
4	*si*	suh	esophagus
5	*wu*	woo	stomach, spleen
6	*liu*	lew	ribs
7	*chi*	chee	liver
8	*ba*	bah	navel
9	*jiu*	joe	lower abdomen
10	*shi*	shuh	anus
11	*shiyi*	shuh-ee	limbs, hands, feet

A single natural number sound is repeated aloud for developing energy in the indicated organ and part of the body. Refer to the example earlier in this chapter in which Linda self-healed her constipation by repeating the natural sound of the number 9 ("joe") to vibrate her lower abdomen.

As another example, if your heart feels weak, you would continuously say the natural sound of the number 2. Say "Ar, ar, ar, ar" while visualizing your heart pulsing with bright red light. Saying the sounds sharply and quickly stimulates your heart cells to vibrate faster and radiate more energy ("ar, ar, AR, AR, AR, AR, AR, AR"). Saying the sounds in a long, sonorous tone produces a gentler effect ("A A A A A A R R R R R, A A A A A A R R R R R . . . "). This gentler effect is the best practice for those who are very sick. Visualizing light in the area at the same time (a mind power technique) promotes energy development.

A combination of two or more natural number sounds is used in power healing for transferring energy from one part of the body to another. Usually, excess energy is directed away from painful or over-stimulated areas to those areas needing energy. The first number in the sequence stimulates the area of the body where excess energy has collected and needs to be dissipated; the second number stimulates the area where the excess energy is to be sent. The Lower *Dan Tian*, located in the lower abdomen, is generally a good place to send excess energy, as it is the storehouse of the body's energy. For example, refer in Chapter 7 to the case of Pat, who self-healed her sore throat by repeating the natural number sounds 1 and 9 ("ee-joe").

SPECIAL HEALING NUMBER, 3396815

The number 3396815 (pronounced "sahn sahn joe lew bah yow woo") is a Zhi Neng medicine mantra or special healing sound. This mantra can vibrate all the major organs in the *San Jiao*. As we saw in the previous section, each individual number of this mantra vibrates and concentrates energy in different major organs. The last number of this mantra is 5 (pronounced "woo"), which concentrates energy into the stomach, which is located in the Middle *Jiao*. Energy flow in the Middle *Jiao* will speed healing in the whole body. The vibrations of this mantra promote energy flow in the whole body. It is an internal massage for the whole body. This special healing number mantra was created by the founder of Zhi Neng medicine, Master and Dr. Zhi Chen Guo.

The number 3396815 has great healing power. Because this mantra promotes energy flow in the *San Jiao*, including all the major internal organs, it can help you self-heal physical, emotional, mental, and spiritual problems. It can also develop the potential power of the brain. You can even use this mantra to heal others, as Roxsane did for her dog.

"My dog Rainbow, a bichon frise, always gets carsick and vomits in the car. She would get carsick even if we went for a little twenty-minute ride," recalls Roxsane. "When I drove to visit my grandchildren, I decided to try the special healing number mantra that I learned from Dr. Sha for Rainbow's car sickness. So I yelled and chanted '3396815, 3396815, 3396815, 3396815! *Hao, hao, hao!* Thank you, thank you, thank you!' Sometimes I was loud, sometimes quiet, and sometimes even silent in my mind, but I chanted the whole time.

"The trip was five hours going and five hours returning. It was snowing that late winter day, and there was almost no traffic, so I was a little nervous, but the mantra kept me focused. Amazingly, Rainbow did not get carsick at all! This was a first for Rainbow. I did not have any vomit to clean up! We got there safely—with no vomit and no nervousness.

"Now Rainbow doesn't get sick anymore. It just occurred to me today as I put her in the car that she doesn't cry anymore either. I guess she used to cry because she got sick and vomited all over the car. But now, driving with Rainbow has become a pleasant experience, for her and for me. Thank you, 3396815. Thank you, thank you, thank you."

You can give other people energy healing by pointing one hand at the person's area of sickness and chanting this special healing number as fast as possible. Do it for at least five minutes a time, several times a day. It will bless your healing results.

Healing Practice
Body Position (Body Power Technique)

Stand, sit, or lie down comfortably. The mantra can be repeated in any position, aloud or silently, wherever you are.

Communicate (Soul Power Technique)

Say "Sahn sahn joe lew bah yow woo, sahn sahn joe lew bah yow woo, sahn sahn joe lew bah yow woo, sahn sahn joe lew bah yow woo, could you help me [make your request for your health or for blessing for your business, relationships, or other parts of your life]?" Say "Thank you, thank you, thank you."

Chant (Sound Power Technique)

Chant "Sahn sahn joe lew bah yow woo, sahn sahn joe lew bah yow woo, sahn sahn joe lew bah yow woo, sahn sahn joe lew bah yow woo" continuously.

Close (Soul Power Technique)

Say "*Hao, hao, hao.* Thank you, thank you, thank you."

Practice Time

Repeat this mantra as fast as you can, for as long as you can.

LING GUANG PU ZHAO

Ling guang pu zhao (pronounced "ling gwahng poo jow") has been one of the most powerful mantras throughout China's history. *Ling* means "soul world," *guang* means "light," *pu* means "widely," and *zhao* means "shining." In total, this mantra means: "The light of the soul world widely shines and blesses."

This mantra can be used by anyone, spiritual and religious people, whatever your religion, and by nonreligious people as well. It can be used by every person because the light of the soul world includes the light of every soul. It can be used for self-healing, for healing, and for blessing every part of your life.

Healing Practice
Body Position (Body Power Technique)

Totally relax your body in any position. Be respectful, very sincere, and honored to chant.

Communicate (Soul Power Technique)

Say "*Ling guang pu zhao, ling guang pu zhao, ling guang pu zhao, ling guang pu zhao,* could you help me and bless me [make a request for your health or for the blessing of other issues]? Thank you, thank you, thank you."

Chant (Sound Power Technique)

"*Ling guang pu zhao, ling guang pu zhao, ling guang pu zhao, ling guang pu zhao.*"

Close (Soul Power Technique)

Say "*Hao, hao, hao.* Thank you, thank you, thank you."

Practice Time

Repeat this mantra for as long as you can per session, as many times as you can per day.

GOD'S LIGHT

In the course of writing this book, I felt enlightened and blessed by a new mantra—"God's light"—which may prove to be the most powerful mantra in the universe. This mantra can be applied for your health, business, relationships, success, and enlightenment of your soul. It can be applied for any request you want to make.

"Like many in today's world, I often get much less sleep than I need," writes Allan. "Many days, my chronic sleep debt becomes acute. One such time, I drove for nearly four hours with two compatriots to an almost all-night meeting. After only a couple hours of sleep, we had to attend a breakfast meeting. As sleepy as I was, I had no choice but to stay awake, because I had to drive the three of us back home nonstop to meet other commitments.

"What could I do? Normally, I would depend on caffeine, but I knew that wouldn't work for the entire return drive. Having been introduced to the four power self-healing techniques, I asked "God's light" to help me stay awake and alert. Then, I sang "God's light" continuously for the entire trip, silently, while my passengers slept blissfully. I had no problems remaining alert and my energy was great for the rest of the day."

Healing Practice
Body Position (Body Power Technique)

Stand, sit, or lie down comfortably. The mantra can be repeated in any position, aloud or silently, wherever you are.

Communicate (Soul Power Technique)

Say "God's light, God's light, God's light, God's light. Could I request God's light to heal my body, mind, and soul, to bless my life?" Request anything you want from God's light. "Thank you, thank you, thank you."

Chant (Sound Power Technique)

Repeat "God's light, God's light, God's light, God's light . . . "

Close (Soul Power Technique)

Say "*Hao, hao, hao.* Thank you, thank you, thank you."

Practice Time

Chant the mantra as many times as you can, for as long as you can, day and night.

In summary, sound power techniques (mantras, natural healing numbers, and other healing sounds) are some of the most powerful in this book. Practicing mantras is very simple and convenient. You can repeat them anywhere, at any time: while you shower, get dressed, ride a bus, drive, cook, clean house, walk, jog, work out in a gym, swim—anywhere! There are no time rules for practicing mantras. You can practice a few minutes at a time or for hours.

By following the principles and procedures behind these mantras, you will experience the benefits for your health, business, relationships, and life. Some people get great healing results and blessings right away. Others get healing results and blessings later. Be patient. Be confident. Don't worry too much about how you're pronouncing the words or sounds. Enjoy practicing mantras for your healing and blessing, and for enlightening your spiritual journey.

You're about to learn the third power-healing technique, which involves the mind and visualization. As you've no doubt noticed, all these self-healing techniques work hand in hand. In the meantime, however, I wish that the mantras bless you well.

MIND POWER

As a flight attendant, Rebecca loved her job and really put her heart into it. So when her airline decided to sell to another airline during her twenty-seventh year of flying, she was shaken to the core. At an all-time low, her security shattered, she suddenly found herself confronting a lot of tough decisions. What would she do? Going with another airline would mean she would probably lose her seniority, which could affect everything from when she worked to her pay scale.

Just when she thought things couldn't get any worse, she had to have surgery to remove all the metal hardware that had been put into the ankle she'd broken eighteen months earlier. Since the surgery would require a lengthy period of recuperation, she wouldn't be able to go on a job interview if she had to. There was nothing to do but submit. She did, however, have one secret weapon.

Having recently completed a healer training program with Dr. Sha, she knew about numerous power self-healing techniques. So immediately after surgery, she visualized a healing light in her ankle. Despite the invasive nature of the procedure,

Rebecca experienced almost no pain. And despite being in a walking cast and on crutches, her energy remained as high—if not higher—than before.

She continued visualizing a healing light in her ankle over the next two and a half months. In addition, she used the One Hand Near, One Hand Far Method to transfer the excess energy in her ankle upward to her lower abdomen, and talked to her ankle. "Strong ankle, perfect ankle, pain-free ankle. Heal now," she'd say. "Thank you, thank you, thank you."

When she went back to her doctor, he couldn't believe how well she was doing, or how fast she had healed. She returned to her job—and to being on her feet twelve to fourteen hours a day—just twelve weeks after surgery. Though no final decisions have been made about whether the takeover will cost Rebecca and her fellow employees their jobs or their seniority, she combats her anxiety with the same techniques she used to control her pain and accelerate her healing. "The power-healing techniques keep me above the stress instead of in it," she says.

A simple body power technique she's recently learned—holding her hands just below her navel with her left hand over her right thumb, and visualizing a thousand-watt bulb in her body glowing increasingly brighter as the energy in her body grows as well—has pumped up both energy and stamina on those long late-night flights. "It really wakes me right up," she says.

She also calls on these same self-healing techniques whenever she gets hit with muscle and joint pain caused by the fibromyalgia that's been diagnosed in fifteen different parts of her body and for the recurrent migraines that used to immobilize her. "You don't have to be a victim to your pain. You can do something about it," she says. "If I use Dr. Sha's power self-healing techniques before the pain gets intense, I can get rid of it in fifteen minutes. That's changed my life."

Creative visualization is a very powerful technique that simply involves visualizing a beam of light, or your ancestors, or God (whatever your belief system) blessing you. At one level, you're simply using whatever image you come up with to focus your mind in order to heal yourself. At another level, visualizing light can help you boost your energy or move and balance energy within your body.

Research has shown the powerful effect the mind can have on the body. In one study, pregnant women were told that they were being given a powerful anti-nausea medication. Instead, they were actually given syrup of ipecac, which in reality promotes vomiting. Talk about a cruel trick to play on women already prone to morning-sickness! Amazingly, however, most of the women reported a reduction in the nausea they felt. "The power of their belief was stronger than the drugs," concludes Joan Borysenko in *Minding the Body, Mending the Mind*.[1]

You can see the power of the mind in action with those research participants who managed to lower their blood pressure through relaxation. "By believing they could lower their blood pressure, patients had been able to do so," writes Dr. Benson in *The Relaxation Response*. "People got better simply because they imagined themselves better."[2]

Patsy imagined herself thinner, asked her body nightly to lose weight by coming into balance, and chanted "love my body." And guess what? She lost twenty-five pounds in a single month. Talk about the power of the mind!

Benson stipulates that you can also see the mind's potential to affect the body in the placebo effect, which we've already discussed. "Researchers had long known that when patients believed they would get better—when, for example, they believed they were taking medicine but were instead taking placebos such as sugar pills—more than 30 percent of them did actually improve. . . . Evolution made [the placebo effect] an innate capability for healing within each of us—a resource that could be effective the majority of the time."[3]

There are even examples of people developing such physiological control that they can survive subfreezing temperatures dressed in no clothes at all, with no negative consequences.

Don't worry, I wouldn't ask you to do that. But I do want you to try something. Stretch your arm out to your side and have someone hold it. Then, using all your might, try and resist as that person pulls it down. Now extend the same arm. This time, however, just relax and visualize a tunnel of light around your arm that stretches through the walls of your home, down the street, to the ocean, and past the horizon. Have the same person try to force your arm down again. Though you're not doing a thing to consciously resist, that person is going to have a much tougher time bringing your arm down to your side.

You can try this same experiment while visualizing balloons holding up your arm, and it will work just as well. Or put your thumb and forefinger together and see how much effort it takes a friend to pry them apart while you resist. Then visualize a circle of energy flowing around your thumb and forefinger and have your friend try again. More than likely, he or she won't be able to do it.

That's the strong impact our minds have on what happens in our bodies. All too often, however, we discount the effects that attitude and state of mind have on the outcome—or even the cause—of disease. Why do human beings get sick and then stay sick? In great measure, it has to do with the worries and fears that trigger, and then result from, the illness. It's natural to be afraid when something bad happens to us. But this kind of negative thinking not only discourages recovery, it also makes a lot of chronic pain and life-threatening conditions worse.

"All thought processes and mental states coexist with related muscular activity and tension," state Dennis and Joyce Lawson in *Five Elements of Acupuncture and Chinese Massage*.[4] So you must change how your think about a situation and force yourself to take a positive stance. "Yes, I can do it," you must tell yourself. "I can get well." When you think positively, results happen.

"Visualization invites the body to specifically imagine the healing where it is required and send the appropriate chemicals and energy to accomplish the task," explains Judith, a hypnotherapist and transpersonal psychologist who works with people who have exhausted other options for recovery. "The body is an intelligent pharmacy, capable of manufacturing everything from carcinogens (cancer-causing agents) like Cortisol to cancer-curing agents such as Interluken II, which currently is being created in laboratories to treat cancer. When we are upset, frightened, or in pain, our sympathetic nervous system creates chemicals that harm us. When we are comfortable and relaxed, our parasympathetic nervous system creates chemicals that help us heal.

"The clients with whom I've used the following power-healing technique, which I learned from Dr. Sha, found that it stimulates something within them that can accelerate that shift toward healing. I remember one woman who suffered from fibromyalgia, which is mysterious in origin and brutally painful. Nothing seemed to give her relief from her chronic pain. When we imagined a golden healing ball, she discovered a wonderful sense of comfort as the ball made its spiral path from the top of her head down through all the areas of sensitivity. It was as if the golden healing ball were touching the pained nerve endings with light and soothing them.

"Best of all, imagining a golden healing ball is a practice I can send home with my clients. Every time my fibromyalgia patient repeated the visualization herself at home, she could provide herself with pain relief and change the chemicals that flowed through her body—with no side effects! And that makes it very magic medicine, indeed."

OPEN AND CLOSED STYLES OF MEDITATION

There are many creative visualization exercises to develop mind power. Buddhist practitioners, for example, visualize different Buddhas appearing in their Third Eye, in their Message Center, or in their lower abdomen. Taoist practitioners visualize the *dan* (pronounced "dahn") forming in the lower abdomen. (*Dan* is the essence of energy. It is the most powerful energy that can accumulate in any one spot in the body.) Some spiritual practitioners visualize the sun rising inside their lower abdomen. Others visualize flowers opening in their Message Center or in their lower abdomen.

There are two methods of *Xiu Lian* meditation, which is actually what focused visualization really is. (See Chapter 7 for a description of *Xiu Lian.*) The Open Style method uses images from nature (such as the sun, moon, forest, ocean, or flowers) as a focus of meditation. An Open Style *Xiu Lian* meditator deeply visualizes or projects an image from nature outside of the meditator's body. The advantage of the Open Style is that creative visualization of natural views stimulates the brain more and develops brain capabilities faster. The disadvantage of the Open Style is that the development of power in the organs is slower. Because the image of nature is visualized outside of the body, the meditator may lose some energy and not feel as strong as he or she wants.

In the Closed Style method, practitioners visualize images of their own internal organs and energy centers. They visualize internal organs such as the kidneys, heart, or stomach and energy centers such as the Third Eye and the Message Center. The meditator concentrates energy on one organ or spot in the body. For example, he or she might concentrate on the Lower *Dan Tian,* a key energy center in the lower abdomen, visualizing a ball of light or visualizing a *dan*, which is a concentration of energy.

The advantage of the Closed Style is that the body gains energy faster, since the focus is inward on the specific energy centers and internal organs. The disadvantage of the Closed Style is that brain capabilities develop slower than with the Open Style, because the Closed Style does not use much creative visualization.

When you practice the Closed Style method, you need to focus your mind and concentrate on a specific part of your body. However, do not focus too much or too long. Be natural. Be patient. Great success takes time. When you focus too much, you will create too much heat in that specific area. This heat will exhaust the body's water, leaving you feeling dehydrated and uncomfortably hot all over. The effect is like boiling water too long over high heat. The water will dry up and the pot will burn. This explains why some people who have practiced meditation for a long time, focusing on one spot, feel exhausted, bored, and unhappy. They do not experience power or peace in their lives. Instead, they feel uncomfortable and unwell. They concentrate too much on one energy center or one organ. They may even quit their practice because they do not get benefits.

Practicing both the Open Style and the Closed Style together is the best way to do creative visualization in *Xiu Lian.* Combining the techniques gives you the advantages of both styles. How do you do this? You can focus an image of nature inside your lower abdomen; using creative visualization of natural views can help you gain mind power faster. When you put these natural views and images in the lower abdomen, the internal organs are stimulated. Your whole body feels stronger and more energetic. That is the beauty of using the Open Style and Closed Style together. You can develop the potential cells of the brain and increase mind power and the foundation power of the organs and the energy centers simultaneously. We strongly encourage the combined Open and Closed methods of meditation for *Xiu Lian* practice.

DEVELOPING THE POTENTIAL POWER OF THE BRAIN

Brain researchers explain there are about fifteen billion brain cells in our brains, but in our entire life, we use only 10 percent of them. The unused 90 percent of brain cells are called *potential* brain cells. How to develop the potential cells of the brain is one of the essential issues for brain research. Awakening and developing the potential power of the dormant 90 percent of brain cells should be a goal for every person willing to develop his or her mind.

There are two parts of the brain. The left brain is in charge of logical thinking, language systems, regular (noncreative) thinking, mathematical analysis, planning, organizing, and analysis of structure and statistics. The right brain is in charge of creative capabilities, inspiration, creative visualization, and functions of the Third Eye. These functions include analysis and summarization of messages, images, pictures, and the field phenomena. Messages can be received in your brain in the form of pictures, images, words, or feelings. Developing right-brain capabilities includes developing the Third Eye, the seat of the ability to receive messages in the form of images.

A number of codes can help you develop both sides of the brain. As we discussed earlier, natural number sounds and other healing sounds can vibrate the internal organs. Different healing sounds vibrate different organs or areas of the body. The founder of Zhi Neng medicine, Master and Dr. Zhi Chen Guo, has developed a set of new mantras composed of number codes to vibrate and develop the left brain, the right brain, and the tissues between them.

To develop the left brain and vibrate the cells in the left brain, the number code is 908 (pronounced "joe ling bah").

To develop the right brain, the number code is 92244 (pronounced "joe ar ar suh suh").

Repeat 908 ("joe ling bah") many times. Chant this as fast as you can. You can chant faster when you are relaxed. Then repeat the chant 92244 ("joe ar ar suh suh") to stimulate the cellular vibration of the right brain. Repeat this many times also, over and over. Chant faster. Remain relaxed.

You can also develop the potential power and capabilities of the left and right sides of your brain at the same time. Between the left brain and the right brain is the band of tissue called the corpus callosum. The number code 01777 (pronounced "ling yow chee chee chee") stimulates the tissues between the right brain and the left brain.

If you want to stimulate the left brain and the right brain at the same time, chant the pattern 01777—908—01777—92244 ("ling yow chee chee chee—joe ling bah—ling yow chee chee chee—joe ar ar suh suh"), repeating it as often as you can. Also, chant as fast as you can, so that the brain cells vibrate fast as well. (See Figure 7.)

Why does this work? The left brain belongs to *yang* and the right brain belongs to *yin*. Chanting the number 01777 vibrates the tissues between the left and right brain. Chanting the number 908 vibrates the left brain. Chanting the number 92244 vibrates the right brain. The more you repeat these numbers, the more you vibrate, stimulate, and develop each side.

"So what does this have to do with health?" I hear you asking. Obviously, if your mind has the power to heal your body, then the stronger your mind, the better. Another way to strengthen your

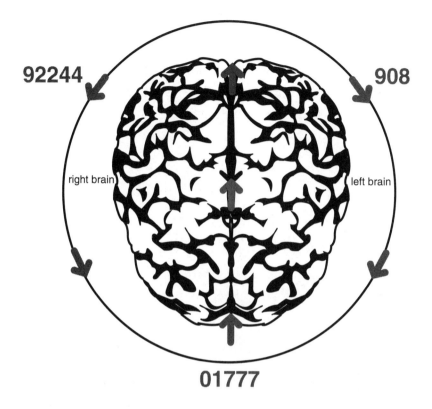

92244

908

right brain

left brain

01777

Figure 7. Number Codes to Develop Left Brain and Right Brain

brain is through the kidneys. That probably sounds odd to you. Traditional Chinese medicine, however, explains that the brain is the ocean of the spinal column. The energy between the kidneys flows downward in front of the tailbone. There are two energy pathways in front of the tailbone. Energy from the kidneys flows through these two pathways into the spinal column and up to the brain, nourishing the brain. That's why the techniques that follow focus on both the kidneys and the brain.

In the mind power techniques that follow, you will also be using body, sound, and soul power techniques to beef up your brain and your brain cells. However, people with hypertension, migraine headaches, a brain tumor, or cancer *should not* practice the following four exercises. People with these health conditions already have too much energy accumulating in the brain and do not need any extra energy there. The rest of us can use as much added energy in that area as we can get.

BOTH HANDS STIMULATE KIDNEYS TO NOURISH THE BRAIN

Healing Practice
Body Position (Body Power Technique)

Place your feet shoulder-width apart. Slightly bend your knees. Contract your anus slightly. Keep your back straight.

Hand Position (Body Power Technique)

Place your hands with palms facing your lower back at the kidney area, just above the waist. Use one hand near and one hand far, with the near hand 4 to 8 inches from one side of your back and the far hand 12 to 20 inches from the other side of your back. (See Figure 8.)

Chant (Sound Power Technique)

Chant the number 9 (*jiu*, pronounced "joe"), "joe, joe, joe, joe," as many times and as fast as you can to stimulate cellular vibration in the kidneys.

Visualize (Mind Power Technique)

As you chant, visualize bright light radiating out from your palms to your kidney area. This will stimulate fast vibration of the kid-

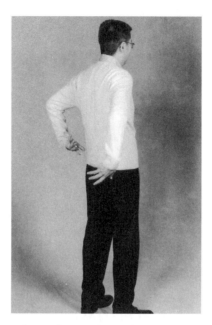

Figure 8. Both Hands Stimulate Kidneys to Nourish the Brain

ney cells and build up kidney energy, which is the foundation energy of the brain.

Communicate (Soul Power Technique)

Say "I love my kidneys, I love my kidneys, I love my kidneys, I love my kidneys. Kidney cells vibrating, kidney cells vibrating, kidney cells vibrating, kidney cells vibrating. Gain kidney power to nourish the brain, gain kidney power to nourish the brain, gain kidney power to nourish the brain, gain kidney power to nourish the brain."

Close (Soul Power Technique)

Say "*Hao, hao, hao.* Thank you, thank you, thank you."

Practice Time

Try to maintain this practice for a minimum of fifteen minutes, the longer the better.

SENDING LIGHT FROM THE KIDNEYS TO NOURISH THE BRAIN

Healing Practice
Body Position (Body Power Technique)

Place your feet shoulder-width apart. Slightly bend your knees. Contract your anus slightly. Keep your back straight.

Hand Position (Body Power Technique)

Hold the palm of one hand 4 to 8 inches away from your body, facing the lower back just above the waistline (kidney area). Put your other hand 12 to 20 inches above your head, with the palm facing your head. (See Figure 9.)

Chant (Sound Power Technique)

Chant the natural number sound sequence 9–1, 9–1, 9–1, 9–1 (*jiu-yi*, pronounced "joe-ee"), "joe-ee, joe-ee, joe-ee, joe-ee," as many times and as fast as you can to stimulate cellular vibration in the kidneys and the brain.

Visualize (Mind Power Technique)

As you chant, visualize light flowing from your kidneys to your head. See the energy like a beam of light shooting out from your kidneys to your head. Visualize the light to be as bright as you can.

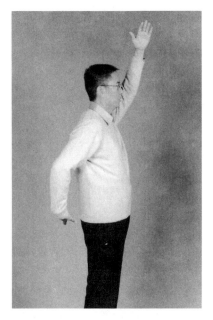

Figure 9. Sending Light from the Kidneys to Nourish the Brain

Close (Soul Power Technique)

Say "*Hao, hao, hao.* Thank you, thank you, thank you."

Practice Time

Ideally, practice this position and visualization at least fifteen minutes at a time, a few times a day.

BOTH PALMS STIMULATE BRAIN-CELL VIBRATION

Healing Practice
Body Position (Body Power Technique)

Stand or sit comfortably.

Hand Position (Body Power Technique)

Hold one hand 4 to 8 inches above the head and the other hand 12 to 20 inches above the head, both palms facing the head. (See Figure 10.)

Chant (Sound Power Technique)

Chant the natural sound of the number 1 (*yi,* pronounced "ee"), "ee, ee, ee, ee," as fast as you can to stimulate cellular vibration in the brain.

Visualize (Mind Power Technique)

Visualize the brain cells vibrating, expanding and contracting, expanding and contracting. At the same time, visualize light radiating in your head, as bright as you can. Keep going, on and on.

Close (Soul Power Technique)

Say "*Hao, hao, hao.* Thank you, thank you, thank you."

Practice Time

Ideally, practice a minimum of fifteen minutes at a time, a few times a day.

PRAYER POSITION TO DEVELOP THE POTENTIAL POWER OF THE BRAIN

Healing Practice
Body Position (Body Power Technique)

Stand or sit comfortably.

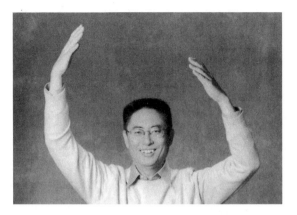

Figure 10. Both Palms Stimulate Brain-Cell Vibration

Hand Position (Body Power Technique)

Hold your hands up in the prayer position, putting your palms as close together as possible without touching. Place your hands in front of your chest between your nipples. (See Figure 6 in Chapter 8.) Keep your eyes slightly open to see your middle fingers. The energy from your middle fingertips will shoot up to stimulate your brain cells and develop the potential powers of your brain.

Visualize (Mind Power Technique)

Just focus on your middle fingertips. You don't need to visualize any light. Gradually you will begin to see light, with different colors, radiating out from your fingertips. Some of you may see your fingers become longer and thicker. Some of you may see many palms alongside your two palms.

Close (Soul Power Technique)

Say "*Hao, hao, hao.* Thank you, thank you, thank you."

Practice Time

Practice a minimum of fifteen minutes, the longer the better. Practice as many times a day as you wish.

Every image you may see in this practice is a response of your Third Eye function. When you see such an image, don't be afraid. This is an excellent response from your right-brain cells, including the Third Eye function. Enjoy and be glad that you can see such a special image.

After practicing the Prayer Position technique for a few days, one of my students in Toronto began to see light about 2 or 3 inches above his fingertips. After ten days of practice, he could see the light shooting out from his fingertips 2 to 3 feet high. After four months of practice, his Third Eye suddenly opened wide. He could see exactly what blockages were inside the body, as well as many other images in the spiritual world. The Prayer Position mind power technique helped him fully open his Third Eye.

This student also gained great healing power. He began to use our One Hand Healing Method. This technique involves standing straight with one hand pointing out to the area where the other person is sick. The extended hand should be about 10 to 20 inches away from the other person. He visualized light radiating in the other person's area of sickness. He used this very powerful yet simple method to help many people recover from their unhealthy conditions.

I've been demonstrating these power-healing techniques since 1990. During that time, I've received thousands of testimonials and success stories from people who are excited to share the great healing results they have experienced using them. They tell of their recoveries from chronic pain, chronic illness, and life-threatening conditions such as cancer. They report on how they experience greater mind power. Many of my workshop participants have gained greater healing capabilities. They have been able to bless their own businesses. Their businesses have improved and their relationships are smoother and more harmonious. They have better family relationships. They get along better with their children.

They've even managed to increase their children's intelligence, whether the kids were in kindergarten or in college. Really! My teacher, Master and Dr. Guo, conducted research in China on one hundred elementary schoolchildren. Some of these children had low grades in math or literature. They could not concentrate or study. The research found a dark brain aura around the temples of the children who could not learn math well. The research also found a dark brain aura around the foreheads of the children who could not learn literature well.

For one semester, the children practiced the Hand Power Technique to Develop Intelligence I'm about to present to you. In just that short time, the school reported big changes in the study habits and capabilities of all the children. They could stay focused longer and had greater understanding of the material. Their creative capabilities also increased. Let me show you how you can practice this hand power technique and get comparable results. Please note, however, that children or adults with chronic headaches, hypertension, and brain tumors SHOULD NOT practice this technique.

HAND POWER TECHNIQUE TO DEVELOP INTELLIGENCE

Healing Practice
Body Position (Body Power Technique)

Sit down in a full or half lotus position or sit with naturally crossed legs. You can also sit forward in a chair with feet flat on the floor and back free and clear of the chair; or stand with feet shoulder-width apart, knees slightly bent, and back straight. Contract your anus a little.

Hand Position (Body Power Technique)

The hand position looks similar to "\ /." The fingers are pointed upward. The hands are close together, but not touching at the wrists and then becoming farther apart at the fingertips. Place your hands in front of your chest. (See Figure 11.) The energy from your hands will stimulate, nourish, and develop your brain.

Visualize (Mind Power Technique)

Visualize the light radiating up toward your head to stimulate the brain cells. When the brain cells are stimulated, potential powers of the brain are activated.

Close (Soul Power Technique)

Say "*Hao, hao, hao.* Thank you, thank you, thank you."

Practice Time

If you are an adult, practice this for fifteen minutes minimum, the longer the better.

Practice with your children for three to five minutes, twice a day. This is enough. Play with your young children and let this be part of a game. It will help your children develop their minds and intelligence.

Why does this technique work? Both hands facing each other

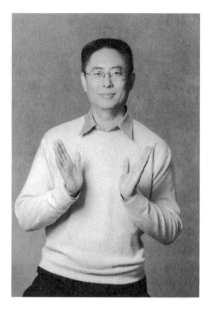

Figure 11. Hand Power Technique to Develop Intelligence

radiate energy back and forth, creating lots of energy. The hand position lets the energy radiate up to stimulate the brain cells and develop the potential power of the brain.

You can practice any and all of the exercises in this chapter as your time and interest allow. If you particularly like one exercise, practice it several times a day and for longer periods each time. If you can find the time, do more than one exercise per practice session. You will gain greater power if you can do two or three exercises together several times a day.

CREATIVE VISUALIZATION EXERCISES

Creative visualization can boost your energy in addition to healing body, mind, and soul. The following seven exercises are mind power techniques using creative visualization for mind power, for energy boosting, and self-healing.

Raging Sea

People practicing *Xiu Lian* (see Chapter 7) want to develop the potential power of the body. They have to do many exercises for the stomach and intestines, where some important energy centers are located. People know that walking, jogging, and weight training are excellent exercises for muscles and joints. What exercises should you do for the stomach and intestines? Creative visualizations and mantras are excellent exercises for these organs, as well as for other internal organs. Why? Because creative visualizations, mantras, and special healing sounds are inner massages for the internal organs.

Let's start with the Raging Sea exercise and you'll see what I mean.

Sit down in a full or half lotus or natural cross-legged position; or sit down in a chair with your back free and feet flat on the floor. Touch the roof of your mouth with the tip of your tongue. Close your eyes and visualize an ocean inside your abdomen and your body expanding as wide as possible to contain the ocean. Visualize that your abdomen holds the Pacific Ocean. The sun is shining. The water is very clean. Then the weather starts to change. The wind starts to blow stronger and stronger. Now it is raining. Visualize heavy rain. Big wind, heavy rain, now a typhoon is coming. Woooooooo. Rain is pouring down. A tidal wave is coming. Thunder and lightning flash in the sky. Visualize all of this happening inside your lower abdomen. Your whole abdomen is vibrating and excited. Typhoon again. Thunder, pouring rain, tidal wave. When you feel the tidal wave, keep the action going for a few minutes.

This exciting situation will stimulate the cellular vibration of your stomach, intestines, and whole abdominal area. Your digestion and absorption of nutrients will be much better. Your foundation energy—critical to good health, stamina, and long life—will be increased tremendously. Follow this pattern and enjoy the Raging Sea exercise:

The water is clear.

The sun is warm.

The view is gorgeous!

Breathe deeply. Feel the energy.

The tide laps gently, from left to right.

The breeze flows, swirling left to right.

Waves are lapping.   The wind picks up.   Dark clouds.

Waves chop. Slapping. Whitecaps foam. Wind Howwwllls!

Wha! Wha! **WooOO! Whoosh!** WHOOSHHH!!

RAIN!!! THUNDER! LIGHTNING!! WIND!!!

WHIP! WHIP! SNAP!! CRACK! ZAP!!! ZAP!!!

TSUNAMI!! HURRICANE!!! TYPHOON!!!!

The whole ocean is Churning! Boiling! *Raging!!*

Waves are smashing! Thunder roars!

S l o w l y **the wind** d i e s

the   rain   t a p e r s

s k y   c l e a r s

quiet

calm

time

time is endless

Five Colored Horses Galloping Up the Mountain

Visualize yourself on a red horse on a plain next to a mountain inside your lower abdomen. As you gallop *up* the mountain, spiral in a counterclockwise direction. Walk, trot, canter, and gallop *down* the mountain in a clockwise direction.

RED HORSE
On a wide open plain
Jump on in your **RED** robes
Walk the horse dinga dinga dinga
Trot Trot *dinga dinga dinga dinga dinga*
Canter *dinga up dinga up dinga up dinga*
GALLOP toward the mountain *dinga dinga*
GALLOP spiraling *up* the mountain *dinga*
higher   higher faster faster faster up up up up
RED horse is SWEATING! STEAMING! PANTING!
SNORT! Whh-ee-ee! MUSCLES RIPPLE !! POWER!
GALLOP OUT ONTO THE TOP OF YOUR HEAD !!!

•

Stop
Rest a bit
Enjoy the view
Sitting on your horse
Turn the horse around
Jump back inside your head
RED horse starts walking, spiraling
Trot Trot *dinga dinga dinga dinga dinga*
Canter Canter *spiraling down dinga down dinga*
GALLOP down the mountain *dinga dinga*
faster faster faster down down down *dinga dinga*
What is that you see in the distance? RED. . . A RED HEART!
GALLOP and RIDE STRAIGHT INTO YOUR HEART

This fast, action-packed exercise develops energy in the five most important internal organs of the body. As you ride your horse and spiral up the mountain, the energy developed in your lower abdomen radiates upward to stimulate your brain. The increased cell activity increases energy in the brain. Coming down the mountain, the brain energy stimulates the internal organs to increase their energy.

Repeat the exercise using *yellow, white, blue,* and *green* horses. Wear robes of the same color as the horses. You and the *yellow* horse will gallop in a counterclockwise spiral up the mountain, pop out of your head, stop for a moment to catch your breath, race back down the mountain in a clockwise spiral and gallop at full speed straight into the spleen (located behind the lower ribs on the left). Similarly, ride the *white* horse into the lungs, the *blue* horse into the kidneys, and the *green* horse into the liver (located behind the lower ribs on the right).

The red horse strengthens the heart; the yellow horse, the spleen; the white horse, the lungs; the blue horse, the kidneys; and the green horse, the liver.

Ginseng Tree Growing on the *Chong* Meridian

Visualize a ginseng seedling growing into a tree inside your lower abdomen.

Ginseng seedling
   In the Snow Mountain Area
Tender shoots reach up
   A trunk grows in your spine
      Young roots spread down to your feet
         Your arms are branches, your legs are main roots
            Standing sturdy, strong, rooted on fertile Earth
Ginseng tree branches grow and fill your head
   Reaching to the Sun—*warm, golden, healing light*
      Bask in the *radiance* as the Sun nourishes your leaves
         Leaves rustle music above your head, *winking* gold
            in the Sun
         Your many fruits feel *light* and rich in the breeze

Take energy from the Earth!
Take energy from the Sun!
Make life force energy!
Send glowing *energy* to all parts of your ginseng tree
Feel the strength, the vitality, the life in your veins
Feel *energy glowing, flowing* all through your body
Nourish all parts from smallest root to topmost branch
All your organs are healthy, strong, and vibrant!
Your roots are bright, shiny, and clean
Your trunk is a glowing golden stalk
Your branches are golden vibrant limbs
Your leaves shine gold and blinding in the Sun
Your fruits are heavenly golden orbs of *energy*
Everything radiates light and energy
You shake with this energy! Vibration!
Feel **STRONG** as the Sun smiles on you
Bend and sway with the Wind
Rejoice in your strength
Relax

The Chinese aptly call ginseng the "man root." Ginseng roots truly look like miniature humans. Because ginseng nourishes *chi* and blood, it is the most revered herb in the East. This visualization is particularly powerful, as *you* are the one growing the ginseng tree inside yourself on the *chong* meridian. Your mind determines how big, strong, and powerful the tree is. As the tree, you are rooted in the Earth. Energy from the Earth and the Sun flow through you, nourishing you. Feel the strength and vitality of the ginseng tree. Draw upon its powerful healing properties as its energy runs through your veins and organs.

Finding a Pearl at the Bottom of the Sea

Visualize an ocean inside your lower abdomen.

There is an ocean inside my tummy
Cool waters are clear blue silk
Smooth as glass
Look deep
Down
D
o
w
n
•
•
•
•
!
Oh!
Look!
A pearl!
A *golden* pearl!
At the bottom of the sea!

Glowing!   Pulsing!
Bright!   Golden!
Beautiful   Perfect
Shining   Pure
Strong!   Brave!
Beacon   Light
How lovely   Just to see
This little jewel!

◆

Concentrate on seeing the pearl at the bottom of the ocean for at least half an hour. It is radiating pure, golden light, and its beauty and energy take your breath away. This exercise directly develops energy in the Lower *Dan Tian* and Snow Mountain Area, and indirectly develops the *Zu Qiao* and Upper *Dan Tian* (Third Eye) energy areas.

Focusing on the pearl stimulates the cells in the Snow Mountain Area, which rapidly develops intense energy. This energy radiates to the brain and helps develop the potential brain cells. Working with the Snow Mountain Area is a safe, easy, and effective alternative to exercises that work directly on the Third Eye.

Three Colored Dragons Playing with a Golden Pearl

Setting: There is a brilliant golden pearl in your Lower *Dan Tian*. Green Dragon is on the left, Blue Dragon on the right. Yellow Dragon has its tail in your Snow Mountain Area, body in front of your spine, head in your brain. They are playing a game called Catch the Pearl.

Pearl jumps up and down.
Green Dragon jumps! Blue Dragon jumps! *Jump jump jump*
Green Dragon sucks in Pearl.
Spits out Pearl . . . *gold dust everywhere*
Blue Dragon *flies* after Pearl. Catches Pearl. Spits out Pearl.
Whoosh!! Green Dragon *chases. Catch Pearl! Spit out Pearl!*
Zooo o o m! Catch! Spit!!! Swoop! Faster!
    Suck! Spit! Suck! Spit! Spin!
      What fun! Wee- ee-e! Hee-hee! Wonderful game!!
The Yellow Dragon's Ecstasy
Oops!

Pearl jumps into Yellow Dragon's tail.

Bump bump bump de bump up Yellow Dragon's tail

> *Oh joy! To have a golden peeaarrrrrl in my tail!*
>
> *Wonderful! Now up my back! Squirm Squirmm m m with ecstasy . . .*

Pearl Glows Blinding Hot! Pulse! Pulse! Pulse! Glow!!!

> *I feel very warm! Purrrrrr!*
>
> *Ahh hh h! Shiverrr r y delight !!!*
>
> *Pearl is in my neck! In my mouth!*
>
> *Twitch! Spasm! Shiver my bones! Ooh h h! How lovely!*
>
> ***Pt-too-ee!***

SPIT OUT PEARL! SUCK IT IN !!! *SPIT! SUCK!*

SPIN! *Pearl spins. Whhrrr rr r r r   whirrrrrr   weee wee*

Pop!

Back into Yellow Dragon's mouth and down his body!

> *Wiggle! Jiggle! Sigh! Lovely! Ahhhh!*

Pop!

Pearl hops out of Yellow Dragon's tail.

Catch Pearl again.

Green Dragon snatches Pearl in his mouth.

> *Mine! Let's play "Catch" again.*

The Green Dragon represents the liver, the Blue Dragon, the kidneys. The Green and Blue Dragons flying inside the lower abdomen increases the energy of the liver, kidneys, and lower abdomen. This increased energy moves and flows through the *chong* meridian when the pearl inches its way up the Yellow Dragon's body. More energy in the *chong* meridian feeds and strengthens all the other internal organs because the *chong* meridian is connected to all the other meridians in the body.

Seeing Yourself in Your Lower Abdomen

Visualize burning fires boiling a lake at the bottom of your abdomen.

FLAMES BURN BRIGHTLY AT THE BOTTOM OF
SNOW MOUNTAIN
    Leaping higher and higher
    Boiling Lake above
YOUR SMALL PERSON
    Sits placidly
    Calmly
    On a lotus flower
    Floating in the middle of Boiling Lake
    Gases explode from the depths
    Whorls of mists tumble and roll
    Water hisses all around
YOU are serene
    Tranquil
    GLOWING!!
    Your body, your organs
    All shine brilliantly
    WHOLE
    STRONG
    HEALTHY
    Clear! Translucent! Pulsing!
YOU are serene
    Sitting on your lotus flower
    In this maelstrom of incredible energy
    Where the Universe ROARS! RUMBLES!
    The water ROILS! BOILS! SPITS!
    The flames CRACKLE!
YOU are serene

The I Ching and traditional Chinese medicine's Five Elements theories are important to this visualization. Water is *yin*; fire is *yang*. Water represents the kidneys; fire represents the heart. Kidney water goes *up* to nourish the heart and gives it *yin*. Heart fire goes *down* to nourish the kidneys and gives them *yang*. The elements, water and fire, nourish, coordinate, and balance each other. When fire is burning and water is boiling, *yang* and *yin* are both excited. *Yin/yang* is changeable at this moment. Your SMALL PERSON sitting serenely in the middle of all this energy is your subconscious mind. See the SMALL PERSON as your soul. The lotus-flower image has special significance and power. Visualizing your SMALL PERSON and your SMALL PERSON's organs glowing with *health*, *wholeness*, and *strength* sends the same message to your subconscious mind, which will translate it into reality in your physical body.

Flashing Images Inside Your Lower Abdomen

Visualize anything you want inside your lower abdomen.

Watch ocean waves ripple in
The sun rising over the mountains blinds you
Pine trees sway overhead
Flowers waving madly
The smiling face of a loved one
Laughing children
Swirling autumn leaves
Rolling clouds of fog
Rushing mountain waters
Golden temples and cymbals
Leaping schools of dolphins
The sky dark with a thousand birds

Mist swirling off the ground in the early morning
A kiss
A puppy's joy
The sheen of oil on a puddle
A glance from across the room
Your home
Rain dimpling a lake
The color of pleasure
Coming home with your newborn child
Wheatfields under blue skies
Dewdrops like crystals in the sun
Volcanoes gushing fiery lava
A gleaming metal structure
Ancient civilizations
Heaven . . .

Visualize anything and everything that comes to mind. See the images sharply and clearly inside your lower abdomen. Open yourself to the feelings they bring. Switch images and scenes as *quickly* as you can. Changing images quickly stimulates vibration of the brain cells and develops mind power very quickly.

YIN MEDITATIONS

The foregoing exercises—the fast-paced, stimulating kind—are what we call *yang* meditation. There is also peaceful and quiet visualization called *yin* meditation. *Yin* and *yang* meditation must be balanced, which makes sense since balance is what we strive for in health and in life. Healing is enhanced by alternating exciting, stimulating, and dynamic *yang* meditation with calm, peaceful, and quiet *yin* meditation.

Enjoy reading the beautifully visual *yin* exercises that follow and practice them with family and friends. Remember to fully experience the beauty of the images, as well as the peace and satisfaction their viewing elicits.

- Visualize a lotus flower opening in your lower abdomen.
- Visualize the sun shining in your lower abdomen.
- Visualize a beautiful garden in your lower abdomen.
- Visualize all kinds of flowers with different colors opening in your lower abdomen.
- Imagine a park located in your lower abdomen where your children and their friends are playing, singing, and dancing.
- Visualize these children filled with purple light and golden light. (Through this visualization you are already sending great healing to your children and their friends.)

You can visualize any beautiful picture or view you wish. But don't stop there. Really steep yourself in the moment. Imagine, for example, that you are standing by a quiet lake at sunrise and taking pleasure in that feeling. Enjoy the nourishment radiating from the shining sun. Feel its energy seep into your body.

The peace and quiet of these moments will also give you healing.

At some moment during the visualization, you may forget your illness because you are enjoying the peace and happiness of the view. You enjoy the view and feel satisfied because your mind is very peaceful.

At that moment, the balance in the transformation between matter and energy at the cellular level changes. Energy blockages are removed and pain is taken away. The practice stimulates healing in your body, while strengthening your immune system. And as it makes you stronger and healthier, it makes you happier as well.

SOUL POWER

As potent as mind over matter can be, you can harness an even greater power to help revitalize your body, mind, and spirit: soul over matter.

What do I mean when I use the word *soul?*

"The soul is the source of the most subtle energies of your being," write Donna Eden and David Feinstein in *Energy Medicine.* "If spirit, as it is often defined, is the all-pervasive, intelligent energy of creation, soul is its manifestation at the personal level."[1]

The Western world uses the term *spirit*, as well as *inner voice* and *inner self*, for the soul. Scientists talk about *messages* (which I'll explain in a second). Are these different things? No, they all refer to the same thing. These interchangeable terms do help us understand the soul's healing potential.

SOUL AND MESSAGE

Just as everything has *chi*, everything also has a soul. In the universe, everything consists of matter. The sun, the moon, stars, the earth, human beings, machines, stones, mountains, oceans, flowers, and animals all consist of matter. Matter is constantly vibrating. Energy radiates out from matter. According to Zhi Neng medicine, energy is tiny matter. The important concept here is that matter and energy are carriers of messages. All matter has a message. All energy has a message. Message is soul or spirit. This means that everything has a soul.

Though most people can believe that all living things—from people and animals to trees and flowers—have souls, they question whether inanimate things have souls. Does a stone or a mountain have a soul? Does a house have a soul? The answer is yes! Each of them has a soul. Does a company have a soul? Does a person's name have a soul? Yes, they do!

Why do some people have great blessings in their life, health, and relationships? Each person and business has a soul. Soul is message. If your company name is not right or your personal name is not right, you may have many blockages along your journey's path.

So it goes with your physical well-being. Human beings are matter. Matter radiates energy out and forms an aura. The aura is the energy field of a human being. Because matter and energy are carriers of messages, we can say that human beings and their auras both carry messages.

If the message of your soul is happy, healthy, and blessed, then you have good health and your personal life is blessed. If your soul is not happy or not healthy, then your health, your personal success, and your relationships are not blessed.

In a word, soul is the essence of your life—in more ways than you might imagine. Just as each of us has a soul, so does each of our organs. Organs such as the heart, liver, kidneys, and brain have a soul? Yes! Every organ has a soul. Every cell has a soul too, because the soul is the message. Scientists today are studying communication at the cellular level. In fact, they are dealing with the cell's soul issues. A cell is matter. An organ is matter. Cells radiate energy. Organs radiate energy. Cells form fields of energy. Organs form fields of energy. Cells and organs carry messages. Those messages are the souls of cells and organs.

Soul power comes from communication with the souls of our cells and organs. Let's revisit our headache example one last time. Using the One Hand Near, One Hand Far Method, you were able to change the density of energy fields and draw the accumulated energy from your head down to your abdomen. Chanting a mantra (using the natural number sound of 1, or *yi,* pronounced "ee", and the natural number sound of 9, or *jiu,* pronounced "joe", in combination ["ee-joe, ee-joe, ee-joe"] vibrated the cells in your head and lower abdomen, moving the excess energy down as well. To bring in the power of the mind, you visualize a bright healing beam of light in your head shooting down to your lower abdomen. Finally, you would talk to your head. Not the way you normally do when it hurts, which for some of you may even involve a few well-phrased curses. Instead, you affirm that you love the soul of your head, and then you ask that soul to help itself.

If that makes you laugh, great! Laughter is a wonderful tonic. But remember how Paul walked out of the E.R. after an acute asthma attack that could have killed him? He talked to his lungs, told them how much he loved and appreciated them, and then asked for them to be perfect—exactly what you should do the next time you get a headache. Repeat over and over again: "I love my head. Give me a perfect head. Thank you, thank you, thank you."

Asking for help from the soul of your head—or any other part of your body or mind—is critical. The act of requesting assistance allows you to relax enough to allow the healing to happen. In essence, by *not* trying to do it all on your own, you open a door for energy to come in.

If you haven't tried using the power of your soul to heal itself, you won't believe how powerful this technique is. But perhaps this next story will give you a clue.

"My life seemed to be wonderful," recalls Nancy. "I had great health, a great marriage, and a great business. Our family home looked lovelier than ever, especially since my green thumb was paying off with the orchids I cultivated. Every Sunday, when I'd go to church, I'd count my blessings.

"Then my husband got sick. When he started attending Dr. Sha's healing class, I went with him. I wanted to be able to assist him in any way I could. Two months later, my husband's health took a drastic turn for the worse, becoming life-threatening. During the next four weeks while he was bedridden, I spent many sleepless nights watching him breathe—thinking each breath would be his last. I couldn't work and my business lost thousands of dollars. I was also involved with a lawsuit and over $100,000 went down the drain. The new vacation home we just bought was in a terrible flood just three days after closing on it. In short, I experienced the worst stress of my entire life. The associated anxiety robbed me of the last little bit of sleep I'd been able to get. At the rate I was going, I was bound to get sick. Not surprisingly, I did shortly thereafter.

"To get well and get over the anxiety I began to talk to my soul. Every day I would set aside time in the morning to become very quiet and talk directly to my soul. I thanked my body, my soul, and all of my cells for being healthy for all of these years, and I apologized for not taking better care of myself and for all the abuse I'd inflicted on myself. I asked my soul to heal itself, and to love itself.

"After being so disconnected with myself and in such emotional pain, I expected this healing process to take a long time.

Miraculously it did not. My soul seemed to open up and say 'Welcome back.' I once again felt connected, at peace, and happier than I had in years. As an added plus I lost thirteen pounds very quickly.

"I quickly began resuming all my activities, taking care of my husband, our business, our homes, all the insurance problems related to the flood, and more. That's when I fell, breaking my wrist and thumb and badly spraining my ankle and foot. I think that God and the Buddhas and saints I had been praying to suddenly said, 'You must slow down. You must take care of yourself first.' I thanked them for the broken bones and laughed at how my soul was teaching me what to do."

YOUR SOUL

A human being's soul is located in the lower abdomen. When your Third Eye is open, you can see what your soul looks like. The soul has its own personality, with likes and dislikes. The soul has all the human emotions, such as happiness, enjoyment, satisfaction, anger, worry, fear, and sadness.

Though the soul exists independently in your body, it's linked with your mind. The soul and the mind communicate in the form of waves. Your soul sends messages as waves to your mind every moment. Everything that your mind deals with in the physical world is communicated with your soul through waves. Many people do not know this. Many people think, "I am deciding about this or that matter." This is not so. The soul is involved in every decision you make in your physical life, whether you realize it or not. Everything in your life is connected. Sometimes your soul agrees with your mind's decisions. Sometimes it disagrees. The final word is with your mind. Your mind decides, "I want to do this. I want to do that." If the soul agrees, things are smooth, happy, and successful. If your soul disagrees with your choice of action and you do it anyway, you may experience difficulties and blockages.

Your soul may be responsible for the things that block you. Unhappiness is caused by disagreement between the soul and the mind. Often an accident is not truly accidental. It may be a warning from the soul world that you should wake up and change the way you are behaving. For example, some people get very upset after a car accident. They get angry and shout at everyone. They may not realize that there may be something wrong in their life that needs to be changed. If they don't change, they may have another accident.

Your soul wants to help you, to support you. However, your soul may have a conflict with your mind. That's why you want to ask your soul to provide assistance with any physical, emotional, mental, or spiritual problems you experience. You may be wondering if your soul knows how to heal your physical body and your emotional or mental problems. The answer is yes! Your soul does know how to heal your body, mind, and spirit. Your soul has great power to do this. That's why it's so important to ask your soul to help your organs, to help your cells, to help you with your emotional, mental, and spiritual problems. Tell your soul sincerely, "I need your help. I do need your help. Could you give me a hand? Thank you."

This kind of communication is one of the most powerful self-healing techniques available to us in the twenty-first century. It can balance the transformation between matter and energy at the cellular level, improve energy flow and metabolism, improve the quality of cellular DNA and RNA, and prolong life.

Since sharing this last soul power technique with tens of thousands of people around the world, many have related wonderful success stories about how these concepts and techniques have helped them recover from chronic pain, chronic illness, and life-threatening conditions such as cancer. Of course, they've also used them to deal with more mundane complaints that still have the ability to make your life miserable.

Rita, a homemaker and mother of three, saw her family's prospects for an enjoyable Christmas holiday growing dim when her sixteen-year-old son woke up one morning with a cold and a bad stomachache. "I need to see a doctor," he insisted. Due to the holiday, she was unable to find one. So instead, she decided to try the power-healing techniques she'd recently learned. First she pointed to her son's stomach, and asked him to do the same. Then she asked him to chant "God's light," with her. After chanting for about ten minutes, Rita asked her son to repeat: "The soul of my stomach, could you help yourself?"

Despite the acute stomach pain and cold symptoms afflicting him, her son began to feel sleepy and quickly dozed off again. Upon awakening several hours later, he announced that he felt fine and asked if he could go play basketball with a friend.

COMMUNICATING DIRECTLY WITH
THE SOULS OF YOUR ORGANS AND CELLS

Why does this kind of soul communication work? Let's review why we get sick in the first place.

No matter what your health problem is, there are only two possible underlying causes. One is excess energy in the space between the cells. The other is insufficient energy in the space between the cells. The effect of both of these causes is an imbalance between matter inside the cells and energy outside the cells. The result is pain or sickness.

When called upon, the soul or the message of the organs and cells can adjust and balance the matter inside cells with the energy outside cells. When there is too much—or not enough—energy in the space between the cells, the cells do not feel good. Cells can be stressed and store tension. Cells have a soul. Cells have a mind. That is why cells can be emotional. Cells may feel upset, angry, sad, depressed, or just unhappy. The cells are like human beings when they get sick. Cellular sickness affects the mechanisms of the entire body as well as a person's emotional and spiritual well-being. So you must talk to your cells, as well as your organs, and ask them to heal themselves.

Let me give an example of how to communicate with the souls of your organs and cells. If you have back pain, unfortunately a very common condition, you'll want to relax your body in a lying, sitting, or standing position. Be as comfortable as you can. A sitting position is best, but if it is too painful, lie down.

Tell your body from your head to your toes, "Relax." Relax your head. Relax your eyes, ears, nose, mouth, and throat. Relax your heart and lungs. Relax your neck and whole spine. Relax from your muscles to your bones. Relax your stomach, spleen, liver, and intestines. Relax your thighs, knees, and toes. Take a few minutes to feel the relaxation. Relax from the outside of your skin to the inside of your organs and bones. From your head to your toes, tell every organ, tissue, and cell, "Please relax. Deeply relax."

When you feel relaxed in one part of your body, say "I thank you for relaxing." For example, if your neck was stiff before and now you feel your neck has relaxed, tell the soul of your neck: "I thank you for the relaxation." After a few minutes, when you feel much more relaxed, begin saying: "I love my back." "I love my back muscles." "I love my bones." "I love the tendons of my back." "I'm sorry you got hurt." "I'm sorry you got hurt by the car accident." "I'm sorry you got hurt by falling down." "I'm sorry you are hurting now." "Can you adjust yourself?" "Promote energy flow." "Take out the energy blockage." "Promote blood circulation." "Remove the stagnated blood." "I'm waiting for you, soul of my back, to do a good job. Please adjust yourself." "You are going to have a perfect back as soon as possible. Every minute, you are healing." "My body's soul, can you give a hand?" "My heart's soul, can you give a hand?" "My kidneys' soul, can you give a hand?" "*Hao, hao, hao.* Thank you, thank you, thank you."

If you are suffering at the physical, emotional, or spiritual level, you can talk to your organs and cells directly. You can ask the soul of the organs and the soul of the cells to give you greater support and better health. The method of talking directly with your organs and cells is message healing or soul healing. It is a very simple self-healing technique. You may notice a change after practicing this technique once. You may see changes in yourself and feel the healing benefits later. Trust your body's soul, your organs' soul, and your cells' soul.

Sometimes you will need to continue this practice for many days to see significant improvement. For example, fractures take time to heal. A person with a slipped disc needs to have the disc put back in alignment. If the condition is very serious, an operation may be needed. No matter how serious your condition is, however, you can talk to the soul of your bones, back, tendons, spinal column, or any other organ or part of your body. Use your mind to send a message to the soul of your back. This is message healing. Message healing is one of the most important self-healing methods. Try it. Feel it. Benefits will come to you.

The following example shows you how to talk directly with your organs and cells. You can use this format to strengthen any organ and to self-heal any unhealthy conditions in any organ or cell.

Healing Practice: Communicating with Organ and Cell Souls
Chant and Communicate (Soul Power Technique)

Chant, with great energy and rhythm, for as long as you can: "I love my liver *hun* (the soul of the liver, pronounced 'huen'). I love the souls of my liver cells. Please help yourselves. Perfect liver, perfect liver, perfect liver, perfect liver. Perfect liver cells, perfect liver cells, perfect liver cells, perfect liver cells."

"I love my heart *shen* (the soul of the heart, pronounced 'shehn'). I love the souls of my heart cells. Please help yourselves. Excellent heart, excellent heart, excellent heart, excellent heart. Healthy and happy heart cells, healthy and happy heart cells, healthy and happy heart cells, healthy and happy heart cells."

"I love my spleen *yi* (the soul of the spleen, pronounced 'yee'). I love the souls of my spleen cells. Please help yourselves. Good digestion and absorption, good digestion and absorption, good digestion and absorption, good digestion and absorption. Wonderful spleen and spleen cells, wonderful spleen and spleen cells, wonderful spleen and spleen cells, wonderful spleen and spleen cells."

"I love my lung *po* (the soul of the lungs, pronounced 'poe'). I love the souls of my lung cells. Please help yourselves. Perfect lung conditions, perfect lung conditions, perfect lung conditions, perfect lung conditions. Beautiful lung cells, beautiful lung cells, beautiful lung cells, beautiful lung cells."

"I love my kidney *zhi* (the soul of the kidneys, pronounced 'djih'). I love the souls of my kidney cells. Please help yourselves. Kidneys function better, kidneys function better, kidneys function better, kidneys function better. I love and appreciate my kidney cells. I love and appreciate my kidney cells. I love and appreciate my kidney cells. I love and appreciate my kidney cells."

Close (Soul Power Technique)

"*Hao, hao, hao.* Thank you, thank you, thank you."

When you are chanting and communicating with your organs and cells, there is no time limit. The problem is that people do not practice long enough. You have to be patient and give your organs time to respond and change.

You can practice in this way with any internal organ or part of the body. At the end of the exercise, please send your sincere and honest appreciation to the organ's soul and to the cells' soul. It is very important to end a practice with hope, confidence, and gratitude. The positive message of "*Hao, hao, hao,*" which means "Get well," "Get stronger," in Chinese, is followed by the statement of gratitude, "Thank you, thank you, thank you." The first "thank you" is for God. The second "thank you" is for the spiritual world, your Heaven Team. The third "thank you" is for your own soul, the soul of your organs and the soul of your cells.

Healing Practice: Liver Cancer

Here is a specific example if you suffer from liver cancer. You can modify this example to help self-heal any unhealthy condition. Be creative. Have fun with the soul communication power-healing techniques.

Hand Position (Body Power Technique)

Place your hands in prayer position (see Figure 6 in Chapter 8).

Communicate (Soul Power Technique)

Say aloud: "I would like to talk to my liver *hun* (the soul of the liver, pronounced 'huen'). I know you are suffering now. I love you so much. Please help yourself. I will help you to get well. I request God and my Heaven Team to help you."

Chant (Soul Power Technique, Sound Power Technique)

"I love my liver *hun*. I love my liver *hun*. I love my liver *hun*. I love my liver *hun*. Liver cells vibrating, liver cells vibrating, liver cells vibrating, liver cells vibrating. Clean liver, clean liver, clean liver, clean liver. Gain liver immunity, gain liver immunity, gain liver immunity, gain liver immunity. Happy liver, happy liver, happy liver, happy liver. Perfect liver, perfect liver, perfect liver, perfect liver. I love my liver, I love my liver, I love my liver, I love my liver. Balance matter inside liver cells and energy outside liver cells. Balance matter inside liver cells and energy outside liver cells. Balance matter inside liver cells and energy outside liver cells. Balance matter inside liver cells and energy outside liver cells.

"Give me a perfect liver and restore my health. Give me a perfect liver and restore my health. Give me a perfect liver and restore my health. Give me a perfect liver and restore my health. Perfect liver cells, perfect liver cells, perfect liver cells, perfect liver cells. Intelligent liver cells, intelligent liver cells, intelligent liver cells, intelligent liver cells. Clean liver cells, clean liver cells, clean liver cells, clean liver cells. Love, care, compassion in my liver cells. Love, care, compassion in my liver cells. Love, care, compassion in my liver cells. Love, care, compassion in my liver cells.

"I love my liver. I love my liver. I love my liver. I love my liver."
Repeat the message. Your liver cells will vibrate.

Close (Soul Power Technique)

Say "*Hao, hao, hao.* Thank you, thank you, thank you."

Healing Practice: Digestive Problems

Here is another example if you have problems with your digestive system:

Communicate (Soul Power Technique)

Say, "The soul of my stomach, can you help yourself recover and restore health?"

Chant (Soul Power Technique, Sound Power Technique)

"I love my stomach. I love my stomach. I love my stomach. I love my stomach. I love my spleen. I love my spleen. I love my spleen. I love my spleen. I love my intestinal system. I love my intestinal system. I love my intestinal system. I love my intestinal system. Balance my intestinal system. Balance my intestinal system. Balance my intestinal system. Balance my intestinal system."

Close (Soul Power Technique)

Say "*Hao, hao, hao.* Thank you, thank you, thank you."

The human body has many organs. Every organ consists of many cells. The transformation between the matter inside the cells and the energy outside the cells is the essential issue for one's health. If this transformation is not balanced, unhealthy conditions will occur. The solution for healing is to rebalance the matter inside cells and the energy outside cells.

We can directly talk to the souls of the cells. We can tell those souls, "I love you very much. I care about you. The souls of my cells, please help yourselves to balance the transformation between the matter inside and the energy outside. Thank you, thank you, thank you."

Talking spiritually with your cells is one of the best ways to balance and improve the quality of your cells. We need to increase the quality of the cells' DNA and RNA. Since every sickness occurs at the cellular level, communicate directly with the cells.

PRAYER

Message healing isn't new. Prayer is message healing. A mantra is message healing. Talking with God, with your Heaven Team, with your own soul, with the soul of your organs, or the soul of your cells are message healings. All these message healings work because messages directly affect and influence transformation between matter inside cells and energy outside cells. The key in applying message healing is to spend enough time with it by using patience, confidence, and trust. It takes time to recover from chronic pain and illnesses or life-threatening conditions.

Actually, prayer is the one of the most powerful message-healing techniques, as many studies have shown. Why? Because God is the highest and most powerful message, soul, or spirit in the universe. Heaven Teams are the next highest messages, souls, or spirits. Message can influence and balance the transformation between matter inside the cells and energy outside the cells. No matter what kind of prayer you use, your prayer sends a message to the Heaven Team of your belief system. The prayer can give you results because your Heaven Team sends a message back to your body, mind, or spirit.

Sometimes prayer does not work right away. For example, if you have chronic pain, a chronic illness, or a life-threatening condition, then you have a serious energy blockage. You have to be patient and remove the blockage gradually.

Another reason? Your Heaven Team expects you to do more kind things and to give more service to people and society. Then your Heaven Team can bless you more. Be committed to share love, care, compassion, sincerity, purity, and honesty with the world—you will feel more blessed. You will *be* more blessed.

"Just who or what makes up my Heaven Team?", you ask. All the souls or spirits in the soul world who connect with your soul and your spiritual journey are your Heaven Team, including your spiritual teachers, special guides, higher saints, ascended masters, angels, and archangels. Your ancestors who care about you are part of your Heaven Team. Don't forget to include the soul of Mother Earth too.

Your Heaven Team is your soul family. In the physical world you have a father, mother, brothers, sisters, wife or husband, children, grandchildren, and grandparents. In the soul world, you also have a family that encompasses the souls that are related to your soul. Because your soul family has been related to you in many lives, it is a much bigger family than your physical, human family. Your soul family loves you and cares about your journey. Your soul family, your Heaven Team, is willing to bless you. When you are sick physically, emotionally, mentally, or spiritually, you can ask your Heaven Team to heal your body, mind, and soul and to bless your journey. They will try their best to help you.

Your Heaven Team grows bigger and bigger as you progress in your spiritual journey. This is similar to a successful person who gains more and more connections over time. If you have done great service to people, society, or nature, you have many souls on your Heaven Team. It doesn't matter what kind of occupation or job you have, or what status you have in the physical world, the more service you give, the larger your Heaven Team will be. You then receive blessings from higher and higher levels of the soul world. Open your heart completely to the universe. Commit to serve the universe. Purify your soul, heart, and mind. Sincerity, love, care, and compassion must be your main concerns. The more service you give, the more blessings you receive from the spiritual world.

Your Heaven Team is very happy to heal your body, mind, and soul; to bring luck to your business and career; to bless your relationships with family, friends and colleagues; and to bless your spiritual journey.

If you have any requests for your health, business, relationships, or spiritual journey, open your heart and soul and talk directly with your Heaven Team: "I love you. I need your help now. I would like a blessing for [whatever you wish to request]." After making your request, totally relax and receive the blessing from your Heaven Team. Feel the energy. Feel the love. Feel the healing. Feel the blessing.

Ask your Heaven Team to give you a hand whenever you are in a difficult situation. Remember, sometimes blessing or healing is instant, but sometimes it takes time. Gradually heal yourself. Heal your body, mind, and soul. Be patient. Have trust and confidence. More and more blessings will come to you. If you don't get relief right away after praying, don't lose confidence. Continue to communicate with your Heaven Team members. They will bless you.

Pay attention to another important issue: If you are sick, asking your Heaven Team to bless you is important, but self-healing is important too. If you have sickness due to energy blockages in various organs and cells, you will get more healing blessings if you are committed to self-healing. It is like a business. A business person does not become successful by just sitting at home and imagining great success. Business success requires lots of effort and work, planning, organizing, marketing, advertising, and communicating. Your personal effort will help your business receive more blessings from your Heaven Team.

In the same way, if you are sick, you can't just ask your Heaven Team to bless your health. You have to make your own efforts to improve your health. If you ignore eating the proper food, getting enough rest, keeping your life balanced, and doing self-healing, your Heaven Team will still bless you. If you take care of yourself, your Heaven Team will bless you more. To receive more blessings, it is also important to practice *Xiu Lian* and to emphasize its components of purity, unselfishness, trust, sincerity, honesty, love, care, compassion, generosity, service, and commitment.

To improve your life, you should first find out the mistakes you have made in your actions, behavior, and thoughts. Then ask your Heaven Team to forgive your mistakes. At the same time, you should commit to not repeating the same mistakes. If, a few days later, you repeat those mistakes, then you are showing your Heaven Team that you are not committed to improving yourself. You are showing that you are not willing to cut the root of the problem. So be aware of this spiritual law: If you don't commit to improve, you will not receive great blessings. Your Heaven Team is waiting for you to improve. The more commitment and effort you make in giving service, the more blessings you will receive.

Your Heaven Team blesses you. Your own soul blesses you.

Healing Practice: Praying to Your Heaven Team
Prepare (Soul Power Technique)

Open your heart. Open your soul. With respect and love for God and your Heaven Team, say your name, aloud or silently, so that the universe may hear you.

Communicate (Soul Power Technique)

"I offer my heart's purity, love, care, compassion, honesty, sincerity, and integrity to my Heaven Team. I have [state your unhealthy condition]. Please bless me and balance the transformation between matter inside cells and energy outside cells in the area of my sickness.

"Heaven Team bless me. Heaven Team bless me. Heaven Team bless me. Heaven Team bless me." Say this over and over.

Chant (Soul Power Technique, Sound Power Technique)

"Heaven Team, please help me." Say this over and over. "I love my Heaven Team. I love my Heaven Team. I love my Heaven Team. I love my Heaven Team."

"Good liver, good liver, good liver, good liver [or whatever organ is in need of healing]. Happy liver, happy liver, happy liver, happy liver. I love my liver. I love my liver. I love my liver. I love my liver."

Close (Soul Power Technique)

Say "*Hao, hao, hao*. Thank you, thank you, thank you."

Though you might not know it, your soul communicates with your Heaven Team in the spiritual world. At the same time, your soul communicates with your mind and your body. Your Heaven Team teaches your soul every day without your mind realizing it. Generally speaking, your Heaven Team teaches your soul at night while you are sleeping.

But you don't only have to rely on your own soul or your Heaven Team. If you are suffering, you can pray directly to God. You can say, "God, I am suffering. I have problems in my physical and emotional life." The technique is to tell God directly, "I am suffering [name the problem]. Will you please bless me and help me? Thank you, thank you, thank you."

Then you'll want to chant "God's blessing" as many times as you can. "God's blessing" can be applied as one of the most powerful mantras.

In doing this prayer practice, it is important to pray long enough. Spend an hour, or at least a half hour, just chanting

"God's blessing." Then you can receive more blessing. Some people pray for only a minute or two. They do not realize that it takes time to receive the blessing at the cellular level.

Healing Practice: God's Blessing
Prepare (Soul Power Technique)

Clear your mind. Have love and respect in your heart. Say your name aloud.

Communicate (Soul Power Technique)

Pray "God, I have a request. I am suffering from [describe your problem]. God, could you bless me and balance the transformation between matter inside my cells and energy outside my cells? Give me a perfect liver [or heart, or whatever condition you want to improve]."

Chant (Soul Power Technique, Sound Power Technique)

Chant "God's blessing, God's blessing, God's blessing, God's blessing . . . " Be ready to receive the blessing. Open every pore of your skin and open your soul to receive the blessing.

"Bless all my organs, bless all my organs, bless all my organs, bless all my organs. God's blessing, God's blessing, God's blessing, God's blessing . . . "

Close (Soul Power Technique)

"I thank you so much for healing my liver [or whatever condition]. I know I am being blessed. Thank you, thank you, thank you."

PUTTING IT ALL TOGETHER

I f you're lucky, you may not have to worry about chronic conditions like asthma or life-threatening diseases. Colds, however,
are a different story. We all fall victim to those. Up until now, the
only option you've had when a cold hits is to try and minimize the
symptoms (with all your remaining energy) and stock up on the
Kleenex. But with these power self-healing techniques, especially
when used simultaneously, you can significantly relieve the common cold.

Healing Practice: To Relieve a Cold
Body Position (Body Power Technique)

Stand or sit comfortably.

Hand Position (Body Power Technique)

Place one hand in front of your chest, palm facing body, about
6 inches away, and your other hand facing the side of your body,
about 10 to 20 inches away. If you have a fever, hold one hand

closer to the center of your chest, and hold your other arm straight out in front of your body, with your fingers pointing away from you. Either way, because you put one hand near, one hand far, energy flows down from your lungs and stimulates cellular vibration inside your chest.

Chant (Sound Power Technique)

Inhale as deeply as you can and vocalize the healing sound "AHH-HHHHH, AHHHHHH, AHHHHHHHHHHHHHHHHH-HHHHHHHH" for as long as you can. If your condition only allows you to chant in brief spurts, just repeat "AHHH, AHHH, AHHH, AHHH, AHHH" over and over. What's important is the vibration created by the sound, which will stimulate cellular vibration and energy flow, clearing the lungs of phlegm and infections, as well as improving your immune system's response.

Now direct the cells of your lungs to vibrate even more by chanting: "Lung cells vibrate, lung cells vibrate, lung cells vibrate, lung cells vibrate."

Visualize (Mind Power Technique)

As you chant, visualize a bright white light in your lungs, to trigger the power of your mind. Visualize your lungs being clear.

Communicate (Soul Power Technique)

Next, talk to the soul of your lungs, which in fact has the special name, po (pronounced "poe"). Say: "Lung po, I love you. Please help yourself. Lung cells vibrating, ah, please help yourselves." Ask God, Jesus, Mary, Buddha, your gurus, your ancestors, or any other spiritual teachers or guides to bless you. Ask for the sun's blessing.

Chant and Communicate
(Sound Power Technique, Soul Power Technique)

Continue chanting "AH, AH, AH, AH, AH, AH, AHHHHH, AHHHHH, AHHHHH, AHHHHHH, AHHHHHHHHH." You can sing all this if you want, and even dance around while you practice this power-healing exercise.

Enjoy your healing—don't be too serious. Sing: "I love my lungs, love my lungs. I love my lung *po*, love my lung *po*, love my lung *po*. Clear lungs, clear lungs, clear lungs, CLEAR LUNGS. I love my lungs. Lungs, please help yourselves.

"LIGHT, LIGHT, LIGHT, LIGHT, LIGHT, LIGHT, LIGHT, LIGHT, LIGHT, LIGHT, LIGHT, LIGHT, LIGHT, LIGHT, LIGHT, LIGHT, LIGHT, LIGHT, LIGHT, LIGHT. Perfect lungs, perfect lungs, perfect lungs, perfect lungs."

You don't have to worry about getting the words exactly right, as long as the concepts are there. And don't be afraid to dance around as if you were in a club. You are. You've just created your very own healing dance. Imagine that your lungs are dancing with you. Sing: "Dancing lungs, dancing lungs, dancing lungs. Increase immunity, increase immunity, increase immunity."

Close (Soul Power Technique)

"*Hao, hao, hao.* Thank you, thank you, thank you."

Practice Time

To speed recovery from the common cold or flu, you'll want to do this three to five times a day, for three to five minutes each time. Just remember to have a lot of fun as you practice these four power-healing techniques simultaneously.

People in all parts of the world have practiced elements of these four keys to self-healing—including creative visualizations, mantras, body positions, and soul communication—without realizing the power of their combination. Although each has tremendous power in and of itself, together they maximize cellular vibration. And as you know, that's what makes your *chi*—or vital energy—flow.

Anita is a seventy-one-year old mother of six and grandmother of two. A real-estate agent for twenty-nine years, she focuses on proper nutrition, stretching, and rest to keep well. So she rarely uses medication, resorting to a Tylenol only in extreme cases. If she gets overtired or doesn't eat well for a while, a couple of muscles on either side of her lower spine tighten up. Occasionally, those muscles will stay painfully tight for a long time. Though this has been happening off and on for fifteen years, she never consulted a doctor or took medication for this. Stretching helped a lot, as did sleeping for an extra hour or two and eating right. So she didn't worry about it too much.

Then came the Christmas holidays, when Anita was dealing with nerve-racking business and real-estate situations. Even though she used all her usual tactics to stay healthy, she nevertheless developed painful tension in her lower back. Because it wouldn't go away, she began to wonder if something serious was wrong with her.

Then, it suddenly occurred to her to try the self-healing techniques she had recently learned from me. Remembering that I said to persist with self-healing for three to five minutes at a time, three to five times a day, she set her kitchen timer for five minutes and sent the excess energy from her lower back to her Lower *Dan Tian* (lower abdomen). In addition, she visualized light flowing in that direction and asked the souls of her lower back and Lower *Dan Tian* to help. She placed her near hand (4 to 8 inches away) over her back and her far hand (12 to 20 inches away) over her lower abdomen (the One Hand Near, One Hand Far Method). Anita chanted "joe, joe, joe" (number 9, for the lower abdomen). She also gave instructions: "Light flows from lower back to Lower *Dan Tian*." Though she did this for the full five minutes, she did not notice any change in her back at that time.

When she got to her office later that day, the other people who worked there were out of town. So she did not disturb anyone when she got out her kitchen timer again for five minutes and repeated the self-healing techniques she had done earlier. She did not notice any change after this five-minute practice either.

Anita's firm intention was to repeat this three more times that day and to keep on doing this for the next several days to see if her back would improve. However, she got busy working and forgot all about repeating the routine. At the end of the day she suddenly realized that all the pain was gone! Much to her surprise, it was also gone the next day. Since then, when the pain occasionally tries to reappear, Anita immediately repeats the self-healing techniques and the pain quickly goes away.

As you've probably noticed from both the exercises and stories that have been presented, practicing these techniques simultaneously isn't difficult. For a few minutes at a time, you're pushing yourself on the four different levels—positioning your body, verbalizing mantras, visualizing a healing light, and speaking to the souls of your cells and organs. Once you get to the edge of that effort, you relax and allow yourself to heal. It's a lot like working out at the gym. You strain your muscles until they actually break down, and then they build themselves up stronger. Of course, my self-healing exercises won't make you sweat, and you don't have to leave your home—or even your desk—to do them. You do, however, have to do them regularly—even religiously.

A healthy person wants to improve his or her health and prevent unhealthy conditions. A person with unhealthy conditions needs to increase immunity and body resistance to restore health. A person with a life-threatening condition, such as cancer, must restore hope and improve gradually until he or she recovers fully. Whatever your condition, many kinds of remedies can be used to help. But never forget the power self-healing techniques, especially the daily fifteen-minute regimen that follows. Whether you're healthy and want to stay that way or facing physical, mental, emotional, or spiritual challenges, the self-healing program I'm about to introduce to you can greatly help by stimulating your cellular vibration and helping to balance the transformation between matter inside the cells and energy outside the cells.

First, let me bring you up to speed on just a few more basics.

ENERGY CENTERS

The five most important energy centers in the body are the following:

- Lower *Dan Tian*
- Snow Mountain Area
- Middle *Dan Tian*
- Upper *Dan Tian*
- *Zu Qiao*

(See Figure 12.)

Buddhists, Taoists, Confucians, and other spiritual and energy practitioners have all paid great attention to at least one or two,

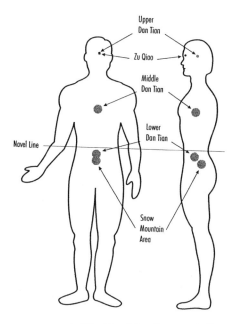

Figure 12. The Five Most Important Energy Centers

and sometimes all five, of these energy centers. After many years of study, I have realized that these five centers are the most important energy centers in the body. Healthy or not, everybody needs to gain energy and power from these five centers to prevent sickness. If you're already suffering from unhealthy or life-threatening conditions, you need to develop these centers first to acquire healing capabilities and restore your health.

Once you learn the location and significance of these five important energy centers, you can practice increasing their power in just three minutes per center. In just fifteen minutes, you will have completed the whole cycle. By including this short regimen in your daily life, you will experience noticeable improvement with your energy, stamina, ability to think, immunity, and quality of life. You will feel happier and more satisfied, and your unhealthy conditions will improve quickly. So, I repeat. Treat this program as an essential part of your daily routine. It's really worth it.

The locations of these vital energy centers in the body are described using a traditional Chinese medicine *personal body inch* unit of measurement called the *cun* (pronounced "tsuen"). To find your personal body inch measurement, bend your middle finger and observe two creases on the palm side of the finger, on either side of the middle section of your finger. One *cun* is the distance from the top end of one crease to the top end of the other crease (not the joint length of your middle finger). Alternatively, one *cun* is also the width of the top joint of your thumb at its widest part. (See Figure 4 in Chapter 7.)

Lower *Dan Tian*

The Lower *Dan Tian* (pronounced "dahn tee-en") is a fist-sized energy center found 1½ *cun* below the navel and 2½ *cun* inside the body. This is the location of the middle of this energy center.

Why do we have to develop this area? This is a foundation energy center of the body. Food gives fundamental energy to the body. The digestion and absorption functions of the small intestine, which is located in the Lower *Dan Tian* area, are improved by promoting the vibration of the Lower *Dan Tian*.

As a result of my years of study and teaching, I have realized that people must develop this area first to gain energy, increase immunity, and build strong stamina to heal body, mind, and soul. I have discovered that people who suffer from chronic fatigue, fibromyalgia, tension, cancer, chronic diseases, and other unhealthy conditions have low energy in the Lower *Dan Tian*. If you want to restore your health, you have to develop the power of the Lower *Dan Tian*.

Because the Lower *Dan Tian* is a foundation energy center, you have to make it a priority in order to heal your unhealthy conditions and to restore your health no matter what your condition.

Healing Practice
Body Position (Body Power Technique)

Begin by sitting in a full or half lotus or with naturally crossed legs. You may also sit naturally in a chair. If you are very sick, you can lie down. You can also stand: Keep your feet as wide apart as your shoulders, slightly bend your knees, and contract your anus a bit. Keep your back straight. The tip of your tongue should touch the roof of your mouth.

Hand Position (Body Power Technique)

With the right palm, hold your left thumb tightly; the left palm should touch the right hand gently. The important point is to squeeze only the right palm around the left thumb with 70–80 percent of your maximum strength. Place both hands on the lower abdomen with the right hand resting on the abdomen. (See Figure 3 in Chapter 7.)

Chant and Communicate
(Sound Power Technique, Soul Power Technique)

Say repeatedly, "I love my Lower *Dan Tian*. Please vibrate more." You can also chant the number 9 (pronounced "joe"). Repeat this natural number sound for one to three minutes, rapidly and energetically: "Joe, joe, joe, joe . . . "

Chant "Gain Lower *Dan Tian* power. Gain Lower *Dan Tian* power. Gain Lower *Dan Tian* power. Gain Lower *Dan Tian* power. Gain immunity, gain immunity, gain immunity, gain immunity. Lower *Dan Tian* vibrating, Lower *Dan Tian* vibrating, Lower *Dan Tian* vibrating, Lower *Dan Tian* vibrating."

Visualize (Mind Power Technique)

At the same time, visualize bright white light radiating (inside your body) in the Lower *Dan Tian*. Use your Third Eye to see the light in the Lower *Dan Tian*. Visualize strongly.

Close (Soul Power Technique)

"*Hao, hao, hao.* Thank you, thank you, thank you."

Practice Time

Practice the Lower *Dan Tian* exercise a minimum of three minutes, but ideally much longer (up to a half hour, an hour, or more).

SNOW MOUNTAIN AREA

The Snow Mountain Area is found by drawing an imaginary horizontal line straight through from the navel to the small of the back. This point in the back is called the *ming men* acupuncture point. From this point, go in one-third of the way along the imaginary line and then go down 2½ *cun* (just in front of the spinal column). This is the middle of this fist-sized energy center.

This energy center gets its name from the Buddhist visualization of a snow-covered mountain in the area. Taoists call this area the Golden Urn. The energy of this area is known to yogis as *kundalini*. Traditional Chinese medicine calls this area the *ming men* area which means "life gate."

The Snow Mountain Area is the most important area in the body because the four most important meridians (*ren, du, dai,* and *chong*) of the body start from this point. Meridians are the pathways of *chi* flow. There are fourteen regular meridians in the body. Every major organ has its own meridian. Twelve meridians connect in a sequence, one after another, to make a circle. Energy moves continuously around this circle.

Healing Practice
Body Position (Body Power Technique)

Stand with your feet as wide apart as your shoulders. Bend your knees slightly. Slightly contract your anus. Keep your back straight.

Hand Position (Body Power Technique)

Place both hands with palms facing your lower back, just above the waistline. Place one hand 4 to 8 inches from your back and the other hand 12 to 20 inches from your back. (See Figure 8 in Chapter 9).

Chant and Communicate
(Sound Power Technique, Soul Power Technique)

Chant *"Hong, hong, hong, hong"* (pronounced "hohng") continuously. This single-sound mantra vibrates the cells in the lower abdomen and lower back.

Next, chant "I love my Snow Mountain Area. I love my Snow Mountain Area. I love my Snow Mountain Area. I love my Snow Mountain Area. Vibrating, vibrating, vibrating, vibrating. Gain Snow Mountain power. Gain Snow Mountain power. Gain Snow Mountain power. Gain Snow Mountain power. *Hong, hong, hong, hong.*"

Visualize (Mind Power Technique)

While you are chanting, visualize bright purple light radiating in the Snow Mountain Area.

Close (Soul Power Technique)

"*Hao, hao, hao.* Thank you, thank you, thank you."

Practice Time

Practice the Snow Mountain exercise at least three minutes each time. Practicing a half hour or more is better.

MIDDLE DAN TIAN (MESSAGE CENTER)

The Middle *Dan Tian* is a fist-sized energy center located 2½ *cun* inside the body, starting from the point midway between the nipples.

From ancient times to the present, Tibetan energy and spiritual practitioners have paid great attention to this area. Tibetan Buddhists named this area the "Message Center" because they believed, and have experienced, this area as the center for sending out and receiving messages from the universe.

In Buddhist practice, one of the most powerful methods for developing the Middle *Dan Tian* is chanting *"Ar Mi Tuo Fuo"* (pronounced "are mee toe foe") while the hands are placed in prayer position just in front of your chest. To fully open your Message Center and to gain great spiritual communication capabilities, you can chant *"Ar Mi Tuo Fuo"* for hours at a time. To practice effectively, it is very important to think of nothing else while you are chanting.

In traditional Chinese medicine, the *shan zhong* acupuncture point is located here. *Shan zhong* is the point where *zhong chi*, the essence of the *chi* in the whole body, accumulates. The essence of the blood in the whole body also accumulates here. If you want to promote the flow of *chi* and blood in your whole body, you must develop the Middle *Dan Tian*. The Message Center is also a key area to develop in order to acquire the ability to converse directly with your spiritual guides in the spirit world.

The following practice shows you how to apply the power self-healing techniques simultaneously to develop the Message Center, boost energy, and self-heal. Focus your mind on the Middle *Dan Tian*. Visualize strongly. Chanting can be done either aloud or silently. Chanting aloud vibrates the bigger cells in the chest. Chanting silently vibrates the smaller cells in the chest. To gain power more quickly, simply chant faster.

Healing Practice
Body Position (Body Power Technique)

The body position is flexible. You can stand, sit, or lie down.

Hand Position (Body Power Technique)

Hold both palms facing your chest with one hand near and one hand far. The near hand should be about 4 to 8 inches from the chest and the far hand should be about 12 to 20 inches from the chest.

Chant and Communicate
(Sound Power Technique, Soul Power Technique)

"*Ar, Ar, Ar, Ar . . .* " is a single-sound mantra to vibrate the cells in the chest.

Talk to your Middle *Dan Tian*. "I love my Middle *Dan Tian*. I love my Message Center. Open Message Center. Please vibrate and radiate."

Visualize *(Mind Power Technique)*

At the same time, visualize bright white light radiating in the Middle *Dan Tian*.

Close *(Soul Power Technique)*

"*Hao, hao, hao*. Thank you, thank you, thank you."

Practice Time

Practice developing this important energy center for at least three minutes and up to a half hour or longer per session.

UPPER *DAN TIAN* (THIRD EYE)

The Upper *Dan Tian* is a cherry-sized energy center located 3 *cun* below the *bai hui* acupuncture point. The *bai hui* acupuncture point is located at the intersection of two lines. One line is drawn from the tip of the nose up over the head to the back of the head. The other line is drawn from the top of one ear up over the head to the top of the other ear.

Taoists refer to the Upper *Dan Tian* as the *ni wan gong*. Buddhists refer to it as the Third Eye. In Western medicine, the Upper *Dan Tian* is in the area of the pineal gland. After birth, this gland gradually degenerates. That is why the Third Eye is closed in the majority of people. Special training and exercises will stimulate the Third Eye (pineal gland) and rejuvenate its ability to see images of the spiritual world. Developing the Upper *Dan Tian* is crucial to developing greater intelligence and capabilities of the mind.

Healing Practice
Body Position (Body Power Technique)

Stand with feet as wide apart as your shoulders. Slightly bend your knees. Contract your anus slightly. Keep your back straight.

Hand Position (Body Power Technique)

Put both hands above your head with palms facing down, with one hand near (4 to 8 inches from your head) and one hand far (12 to 20 inches from your head). (See Figure 10 in Chapter 9.)

Chant and Communicate
(Sound Power Technique, Soul Power Technique)

Chant "*Yi, yi, yi, yi . . .*" (pronounced "ee"). This single-sound mantra vibrates the cells of the brain.

"*Yi, yi, yi, yi.* I love my Third Eye. I love my Third Eye. I love my Third Eye. I love my Third Eye. Open Third Eye. Open Third Eye. Open Third Eye. Open Third Eye. Third Eye vibrating, Third Eye vibrating, Third Eye vibrating, Third Eye vibrating. I want to open Third Eye. I want to open Third Eye. I want to open Third Eye. I want to open Third Eye. Please help me. Please help me. Please help me. Please help me. Gain Third Eye power, gain Third Eye power, gain Third Eye power, gain Third Eye power. *Yi, yi, yi, yi . . .*"

Visualize (Mind Power Technique)

At the same time, visualize bright white light radiating in your Third Eye.

Close (Soul Power Technique)

"*Hao, hao, hao.* Thank you, thank you, thank you."

Practice Time

Practice the Upper *Dan Tian* exercise for at least three minutes. To open the Third Eye, you must practice every day for a half hour or more per session. It may take many days, even months, to open the Third Eye.

ZU QIAO

The *Zu Qiao* (pronounced "zoo chow") is a cherry-sized energy center found just inside the bone cavity behind the *yin tang* acupuncture point (midpoint between the eyebrows).

The *Zu Qiao* is a very important energy center for brain power. For developing mind power, the potential capabilities of the brain, and the healing power of the brain, you must develop the *Zu Qiao* area.

Healing Practice
Body Position (Body Power Technique)

Stand with feet as wide apart as your shoulders. Bend your knees, contract your anus slightly, and keep your back straight.

Hand Position (Body Power Technique)

Hold your hands in front of your forehead, one hand near, one hand far, with both palms facing the point between the eyebrows. Keep the near hand 4 to 8 inches from your forehead and the far hand 12 to 20 inches from your forehead.

Chant and Communicate
(Sound Power Technique, Soul Power Technique)

Chant *"Weng, weng, weng, weng . . . "* (pronounced "wung").

"*Zu Qiao* vibrating, *Zu Qiao* vibrating, *Zu Qiao* vibrating, *Zu Qiao* vibrating. Gain mind power, gain mind power, gain mind power, gain mind power. Gain potential capabilities of the brain, gain potential capabilities of the brain, gain potential capabilities of the brain, gain potential capabilities of the brain. *Zu Qiao* radiating, *Zu Qiao* radiating, *Zu Qiao* radiating, *Zu Qiao* radiating. Gain *Zu Qiao* power, gain *Zu Qiao* power, gain *Zu Qiao* power, gain *Zu Qiao* power. *Weng, weng, weng, weng.*

"I love my *Zu Qiao*. I love my *Zu Qiao*. I love my *Zu Qiao*. I love my *Zu Qiao*. Develop *Zu Qiao*, develop *Zu Qiao*, develop *Zu Qiao*, develop *Zu Qiao*."

Visualize (Mind Power Technique)

While you are chanting, visualize bright white light radiating in your *Zu Qiao* area.

Close (Soul Power Technique)

"*Hao, hao, hao.* Thank you, thank you, thank you."

Practice Time

Practice the *Zu Qiao* exercise for at least three minutes. If you can do a half hour or more, that is even better.

This is foundation healing. If you're in good health, practice each of the exercises related to these vital energy centers for three minutes a day (for a daily total of fifteen minutes) to maintain good health and to prevent illness. For more serious conditions, practice more times a day and spend at least fifteen minutes on each energy center. To develop spiritual communication capabilities, such as opening the Third Eye to see the soul world and opening the Message Center to converse with the soul world, long and devoted practice is required. Practice at least a half hour at a time on the Third Eye and Message Center.

This regimen is a vital part of building your self-healing power. It is as important for self-healing as food, water, and air are for life. I wish I could tell you that by following this program every day, you'll never be sick or in pain again. I can't. I *can* promise you that energy-building techniques like those you just read about and the ones that follow will help keep you healthier and relieve stress and hypertension (two of the main culprits behind so many of our problems). Other even more serious conditions will be relieved as well. As I hope you'll soon see (if you haven't started in already), transferring energy by eliminating blockages in the body can help you heal some critical conditions faster and more effectively than without power self-healing. That's certainly what Dr. Pierre-Louis Faudry, a psychiatrist from Ottawa, discovered:

"Dr. Sha's power self-healing methods have been helping my wife, Carmen, and me tremendously for seven years, where other methods have had only limited or no success.

"In 1982 Carmen began experiencing some health problems. Then her conditions worsened. Her main problems were skin eruptions; extreme fatigue (she could not work for fifteen minutes without resting for hours); fluctuating body temperature with the sensation of ice in her bones; inflammation; redness and a blocked sensation in her ankles and wrists; cramps in her hands; dry skin with an intense burning sensation; different colors in her skin; dizziness; migraines; loss of memory; blurred vision; lack of eye coordination; instability while walking; and lack of overall coordination.

"Carmen was very worried. The whole family was very concerned. Carmen consulted with many specialist doctors, including a rheumatologist, internal medicine specialist, gynecologist, neurologist, dermatologist, and opthamologist. Many laboratory tests and other explorations were done. The consultations and explorations did not determine the causes of Carmen's troubles, nor did they point her in the direction of a solution.

"In 1988 Carmen consulted with an acupuncturist who helped her gain some energy and who suggested that she take tai chi lessons to further stabilize and increase her energy. Then Carmen met a Chinese master who taught her a variety of qigong healing exercises. The exercises helped Carmen feel less cold. However, her energy was still unstable, and she was still experiencing other disturbing symptoms.

"In 1994, Carmen and I and our daughter met Dr. Sha. This was the beginning of a major improvement in Carmen's functioning. With patience, regularity, and discipline, she practiced the Standing *Dong Yi Gong* exercises [which you're about to learn] every day. Within a few weeks, her energy was much better balanced. Progressively, symptoms such as migraines, fatigue, dizziness, and unstable temperature improved, then disappeared. Her energy level was much greater. Carmen could actually feel the energy moving along specific pathways within her body, generating a blissful sensation. All of the subsequent meetings and classes with Dr. Sha have contributed to the further development of Carmen's energy.

"Every day, we thank Dr. Sha and we pray to God to bless him and help him spread these self-healing techniques successfully all over the world. These are priceless gifts that Dr. Sha is offering to the general public. It is such a generous act to make accessible these powerful healing methods, which in the past were taught to only a privileged few."

STANDING DONG YI GONG

Like most of the practices in this book, the standing *Dong Yi Gong* exercises (which literally means "using thinking exercises") use special standing and hand positions (body power), mantras and special healing sounds (sound power), creative visualization (mind power), and communication (soul power) to quickly and safely develop energy in your body, mind, and soul. These exercises will also help balance your body's energy when you are sick.

Practicing this sequence of exercises stimulates the mind and develops power and energy in the five most important energy centers of the body. You may use it as a supplement to the self-healing program just introduced. Though the entire sequence can be performed in fifteen minutes to a half hour—spending more time will yield greater benefits. So repeat these powerful exercises as often as you like—and enjoy!

Standing *Dong Yi Gong* Exercise Sequence
Key Steps

- Be relaxed.

- Where the exercises indicate hand positions (body power techniques) with one hand near and one hand far, hold the near hand 4 to 8 inches from the body and the far hand 12 to 20 inches from the body.

• Keep your fingers level. Do not point them away from the body or downward.

• Repeat the indicated healing sounds (sound power techniques) aloud or silently, as fast as you can.

• Concentrate on visualizing (mind power technique) the indicated area glowing with bright white light.

• Start with the Basic Position for Standing *Dong Yi Gong* as described below.

Basic Position

Stand comfortably.

Keep your feet together.

Bend your knees slightly.

Keep your hands at your sides.

Contract your anus slightly.

Keep your back straight.

Smile slightly.

Touch the tip of your tongue to the roof of your mouth.

Close your eyes slightly.

Relax.

Position 1: Opening to Receive

Move your left foot to the side (feet shoulder-width apart).

Place your right palm 3 inches above the navel, facing upward.

If you have hypertension, a headache, a brain tumor, or cancer, then place your right palm facing down.

Place your left palm 3 inches below the navel, facing upward.

Relax.

You will recognize this as the Open *San Jiao* Body Power Technique from Chapter 7. Hold this position for a few minutes.

Position 2: Energizing the Lower Dan Tian

Put your feet together again (move your left foot back to the right foot).

Place both palms over the navel.

Visualize a light bulb in the Lower *Dan Tian* area. See it burning at 40 watts, 60 watts, 100 watts, 500 watts, becoming brighter and brighter; 1,000 watts, 10,000 watts! Imagine an explosion of light. The whole abdomen shines and glows! It radiates brilliant, clear white light.

Relax.

Bring your hands down to your sides.

Position 3: Energizing the Zu Qiao and the Upper Dan Tian

Raise the arms straight out from your sides to shoulder level, palms facing forward.

Turn your palms up, and bring your arms straight out in front of you.

Bend your elbows and bring your palms to face you.

Hold your palms facing the head area or the Upper *Dan Tian*, with one hand near, one hand far.

Communicate: "I love my *Zu Qiao* and Upper *Dan Tian*. Gain power in my *Zu Qiao* and Upper *Dan Tian*."

Visualize light glowing in the *Zu Qiao* and/or the Upper *Dan Tian*.

Visualize bright white light vibrating inside your head. Every brain cell is vibrating fast and excited. See the whole brain as full of bright, clear light and radiating energy.

At the same time, chant *"Weng, weng, weng, weng . . . "* (pronounced "wung") or the natural sound of the number 1, *"Yi, yi, yi, yi . . . "* (pronounced "ee").

Position 4: Energizing the Middle Dan Tian

Move both palms down to face the Middle *Dan Tian*, with one hand near, one hand far.

Communicate: "I love my Middle *Dan Tian*. Open my Message Center."

Visualize brilliant light radiating in the Middle *Dan Tian* (the lungs and the heart).

At the same time, chant *"Ar, ar, ar, ar . . . "* This sound will directly vibrate your lungs, your bronchial tubes, and your heart.

See the Middle *Dan Tian* vibrating with bright, clear light.

See your heart and lungs as very clean and healthy. When you have very strong energy in these parts, it will help you heal shortness of breath and heart problems.

Position 5: Re-energizing the Lower Dan Tian

Move your hands down to face the lower abdomen with one hand near, one hand far.

Communicate: "I love my Lower *Dan Tian*. Gain Lower *Dan Tian* power."

Repeat *"Hong, hong, hong, hong . . . "* (pronounced "hohng") or the natural sound of the number 9, *"Jiu, jiu, jiu, jiu . . . "* (pronounced "joe").

Visualize an ocean inside your lower abdomen. The ocean is churning, foaming, roaring! Let the fresh ocean waters cleanse your whole abdomen. Let it cleanse your stomach, intestines, liver, spleen, urinary bladder, and urethra.

Position 6: Invoking Higher Powers

Place your hands in the prayer position.

Slightly close your eyes and focus on your fingertips.

Repeat the Zhi Neng medicine special healing number 3396815, *san san jiu liu ba yao wu*, pronounced "sahn sahn joe lew bah yow woo," many times and rapidly.

Position 7: Absorbing Energy from the Sun

Move your left foot to the side again (feet shoulder-width apart).

Hold your palms over your head, with one hand near, one hand far.

Visualize sunlight shining down on you. It shines through you from your head and throughout your whole body down to your feet. The sunshine makes your whole body very warm, bright, and transparent.

Move your arms apart slightly and tilt your hands to face the top of your head.

Continue to imagine sunlight shining through your body. If any part of your body has a problem, imagine that part as bright, shiny, clean, and healthy.

Position 8: Horse-Riding Stance

- Move your hands back down to the prayer position.
- Squat down slowly, keeping your back straight and your thighs horizontal (parallel to the ground).
- Keep your heels and feet flat on the floor.
- Run your tongue over your teeth and around the inside of your mouth to gather saliva.
- Swallow and visualize the saliva going down to the Lower *Dan Tian*. Repeat three times.
- Slowly rise to the Basic Position.

Position 9: Returning to the Lower Dan Tian

Place both palms facing your lower abdomen, with one hand near, one hand far.

Communicate: "I love my Lower *Dan Tian*. Gain Lower *Dan Tian* power."

Visualize the whole abdomen glowing from the inside with bright, clear light.

Silently repeat *"Hong, hong, hong, hong . . . "* (pronounced "hohng").

Position 10: Visiting the Snow Mountain Area

Place both hands behind you with the palms facing the Snow Mountain Area, with one hand near, one hand far.

Communicate: "I love my Snow Mountain Area. Gain Snow Mountain power."

Visualize a snow-covered mountain in the Snow Mountain Area. Imagine a very hot, strong sun shining on the mountain. The snow is melting, and energy in the form of steam flows to any part of your body that you wish to nourish or heal.

Lower your hands to your sides with the palms facing your body.

Position 11: Energizing the Upper, Middle, and Lower Dan Tian Areas

Hold your palms facing the Upper *Dan Tian* or head, with one hand near, one hand far.

Communicate: "I love my Upper *Dan Tian*. Gain Upper *Dan Tian* power."

Inhale deeply and repeat *"Weng, weng, weng, weng . . . "* (pronounced "wung") continuously as you exhale. When you say *"weng,"* visualize the whole brain glowing with clear red light.

Move your palms to face the Middle *Dan Tian* or chest.

Communicate: "I love my Middle *Dan Tian*. Gain Middle *Dan Tian* power."

Inhale deeply and repeat *"Ah, ah, ah, ah"* continuously as you exhale. When you say *"ah,"* visualize the whole chest glowing with clear white light.

Now move your palms to face the Lower *Dan Tian* or lower abdomen.

Communicate: "I love my Lower *Dan Tian*. Gain Lower *Dan Tian* power."

Inhale deeply and repeat *"Hong, hong, hong, hong . . . "* (pronounced "hohng") continuously as you exhale. When you say *"hong,"* visualize the whole abdomen glowing with clear blue light.

Repeat many times.

Position 12: Healing with a Golden Ball in the Abdomen

Place both palms on your navel.

Bring your feet together.

Imagine bright, cosmic light shining down on you from above. Feel the energy flowing through your head down to your Lower *Dan Tian*.

From below, imagine bright light (the energy of the earth) flowing up through your feet to your Lower *Dan Tian*.

Visualize a golden-light healing ball spinning inside your lower abdomen. Concentrate on the ball, and enjoy its beautiful, powerful, clear gold light. Spin it. Spin it faster, faster, faster . . . .

Lower your hands to your sides, with palms facing the body.

Relax.

Do you feel the energy flow as your self-healing efforts work more and more effectively?

But perhaps you're painfully eager to go beyond bolstering your immune system. If the word *pain* strikes an all too familiar chord, stay tuned. That's next.

Pain Away

Pain—from a silly paper cut or hangnail to chronic suffering—is one of the most debilitating experiences life has to offer. As too many of you know all too well, pain has a way of taking over your whole existence, dictating everything from what you focus on (pain!) to what you can do. And all too often pain-relief medication doesn't really take the pain away fully. It may dull it somewhat (dulling you in the process), but it doesn't really reduce it, and it sure doesn't eliminate it.

Enter the power self-healing techniques. By applying them simultaneously, you can control pain of all sorts and potentially even get rid of it altogether.

"On a personal level, Zhi Neng medicine self-healing has come to mean, 'Anything that improves my connection to all of life, the universe, and the Tao, including the ways to heal the body, mind, and spirit,'" says a grateful Steven. "When Dr. Sha taught his first practitioner-level course on Zhi Neng medicine healing and self-healing, I was the first graduate of that program. When he taught acupuncture, energy massage, and Zhi Neng medicine herbs, I was also a part of those programs. Whatever Dr. Sha had to teach,

I was ready to learn, not just the techniques, but more important, the principles. Since meeting him, I have tried to put into practice advice he commonly gives students, 'Have an open mind; then you can learn with creativity and flexibility.'

"I have a background in teaching and printmaking. Being open, creative, and flexible are ways of being that I know from teaching and making art. So it was a very natural flow to connect my foundation in the visual arts with the Zhi Neng medicine healing arts. And that has helped me—and those around me—more than I can say.

"During a beginners' workshop we were taught simple techniques for relieving neck pain. I placed my near hand close to where my neck was stiff and my far hand facing my lower abdomen. I repeated the natural number sounds 1 and 9, *'yi jiu, yi jiu"* (pronounced "ee-joe"), and at the same time visualized light flowing down from my neck to my Lower *Dan Tian.*

"The following week, my friend Jock had a very stiff and painful neck. I showed him the techniques and how to use hand position, sounds, and visualization. In less than a minute he was turning his head freely and said, 'Steven, you won't believe this! I'm almost completely better!' Of course I believed him, as I had experienced the same simple, powerful good results just the week before. This was the start of my healing career.

"Since then, I have adopted the Zhi Neng medicine methods as my healing foundation. Recently, Ruth, a friend of a friend, was in the emergency ward of the hospital for whiplash from a car accident. We went immediately to assist her. She was in shock and her vital signs were being monitored. Her heart rate was very high, at 120. We set to work with the four self-healing power systems and were able to see her heart rate drop to under 100 immediately. Ruth later said to me upon returning home, 'The touch of your hand and receiving Zhi Neng medicine was the most healing aspect of my hospital stay.' She felt a gentle touch, but experienced a deep healing.

"More recently, Jane woke up with a painful headache and painful tension in her jaw, neck, shoulders, and back, top to bottom. Later that morning she experienced total relief with the four keys to power healing.

"Again, all I did was apply the four power-healing techniques, and her headache immediately dissipated. Within fifteen minutes, not only was her headache completely gone, so were her other pains. She walked away feeling energized during the day and had a restful sleep that night. It is very inspiring and humbling to be able to bring relief to others so quickly with such simple methods."

Back problems are another common affliction these days. If your back has ever gone out, you know exactly how crippling that can be. Suddenly all you can do is lie flat with your knees on a pillow and pray that you won't have to sneeze (thereby wrenching your back) or go to the bathroom (which would require you to move). But there is help. I know because I used power self-healing techniques on myself when I hurt my own back seriously.

Healing Practice: Back Pain
Body Position (Body Power Technique)

Stand or sit comfortably.

Hand Position (Body Power Technique)

Using the One Hand Near, One Hand Far Method, place one hand behind your back, with your palm facing the painful area about 4 to 8 inches away. Keep your other hand behind your back as well, but hold it 10 to 20 inches away from you, with the palm turned in. (If both sides of your back hurt, then you'll want to alternate your hands every three minutes, moving the near hand away to become the far hand and the far hand closer to become the near hand.) This will transfer the excess energy from the painful area to other parts of your body where it can do some good.

Chant (Sound Power Technique)

Chant the Chinese words for 9 (pronounced "joe") to vibrate your lower abdomen and 6 (pronounced "lew") to vibrate the area by your rib cage. Put together, it sounds like "joe-lew." Repeat these natural number sounds over and over again.

Visualize (Mind Power Technique)

Close your eyes and visualize a radiant, healing light dissolving the energy blockage in your back that is causing you pain. Next visualize cellular vibration in that painful area. Remember to keep your One Hand Near, One Hand Far position.

Communicate (Soul Power Technique)

Finally, ask your body to provide you with relief. "The soul of my back, the soul of my hands, please work together to give me a perfect back." You can also chant the word "Light" as quickly as you can. After about five minutes, close with, "I love my back, love my back, perfect back, perfect back."

Close (Soul Power Technique)

"Hao, hao, hao. Thank you, thank you, thank you."

Practice Time

Practice about five minutes at a time, several times a day as needed.

Of course, other kinds of pain can be equally crippling.

Marie, a nurse and president of the Institute of Healing Arts and Sciences, pulled a muscle in her chest while lifting and repositioning a two-hundred-pound patient. Suddenly turning her body in any direction, no matter how slight, would cause sharp pain. Even trying to breathe normally was quite painful. Breathing deeply was out of the question.

She probably should have excused herself from work right away, but she suffered through the rest of her shift in a state of agony. Driving home that night proved no easier. She couldn't find a comfortable sitting position. Turning her head to watch traffic was difficult and downright painful.

"Then the fog caused by my pain lifted ever so slightly, just enough for me to recall one of the great mantras that I learned from Dr. Sha," she recalls. "I started chanting *'Weng ar hong'* for about ten minutes. To my surprise, I could breathe freely, turn my head, and move my body without pain.

"In my twenty years of experience in integrative medicine, I have never encountered self-healing tools as simple and practical—and as powerful and effective—as his four power self-healing techniques."

Whether your daily routine involves manual labor or not, life these days isn't kind to us when it comes to body mechanics. In an era when modern technology is supposed to be making things easier, most of us have jobs that involve repetitive motions or postures that strain our bodies in ways that take a toll. No wonder the numbers of people suffering from carpal tunnel syndrome are going through the roof! Though Western medicine has not found an effective way to treat the people with this condition, there is hope.

Frances, in her late forties, has been an administrative analyst for a teaching hospital for about five years. Her job involves entering a lot of data, so she works on the computer about 80 percent of her work day. This has led to a problem in her wrist, which started about three or four years ago. She tried to ignore the pain at first. When it continued to worsen, she went to the doctor and was told she had tendonitis.

"It was not that bad yet, but I didn't want to let it go too long," recalls Frances. The doctors, however, didn't do much for her, especially since Frances had made clear her preference for using gentler forms of healing rather than taking drugs. Their one solution was to send Frances to a hand therapist, who worked on her with massage and taught her some stretching exercises. Though Frances would do the exercises and take breaks as recommended, this therapy only gave her temporary relief; the pain would come back. Still, she refused to take any drugs for the pain.

Finally she tried my power self-healing techniques—and they worked. Now when she starts to feel pain in her wrist, she stops what she's doing, points to her wrist, visualizes bright light in her wrist, asks the soul of her wrist to help itself, sends love to her wrist, and chants "God's Light" and "Golden Healing Ball." In less than a minute the pain dissipates and Frances can continue working. This works for her every time.

"The pain just goes away," she says. "That's really amazing to me."

Only lately has she realized that the pain that threatened to limit her ability to work has simply disappeared. "I don't have that problem anymore," she says. "It just sort of went away. I don't feel that aching pain in there the way I was feeling it just six months ago."

Frances became such a convert that she has also used these techniques to help her mom. Her mother had been plagued with chronic foot pain for about a year. She complained that it was really painful and that when she walked she had to stop and massage her foot to relieve the cramping, but the pain would always come back. The doctor couldn't provide any explanation for this pain. He simply gave her an orthotic to wear. It helped a bit, but the pain never completely went away.

So Frances tried applying the four power self-healing techniques. She visualized her *yin* companions (guardian angels) and her healing Buddha, to whom she feels very close, and asked for their help. She told her mother to relax and pray with her as she pointed her fingers at her mother's foot. Frances asked for the soul of Mom's foot to help itself and also for the assistance of the souls of Mom's tendons, bones, muscles, tissues, skin, and blood. Asking for a perfect, healthy, beautiful foot for her mother, she began to chant "God's Light" and the natural healing sound of the number 11.

A couple of minutes later her mother felt a tingling sensation in her foot and the pain diminished substantially. She hasn't complained about her foot since.

Frances and her mother suffered from chronic pain. What's chronic pain? Chronic pain is defined as pain that lasts for at least a year. Just as with illness, it's caused by an energy imbalance that has not been released or corrected. Unless it's dealt with, the imbalance can have even more painful ramifications.

"I never dreamed I would ever consider a quick end to my life," says Mimi, a youthful, vibrant homemaker in her fifties. "But there I was, entertaining the thought in the months before I met Dr. Sha. Much of my body had been severely traumatized by a physical therapist who was treating me for a frozen left shoulder. Too much pressure and strong massage were applied to my sternum and chest for too long a period. This trauma, coupled with pulley exercises, tore my body apart internally. I felt as though I had been hit by a truck, assaulted, and my insides smashed, ripped, and misaligned.

"The debilitating pain multiplied. Soon my chest, neck, throat, spine, shoulders, diaphragm, ribs, eyes, guts, kidneys, groin, and legs hurt as well! My health deteriorated rapidly. Adding to the injuries, the harm inflicted seemed malicious and intentional. The therapist never returned my calls or my doctors'. My doctors were unable to provide much help. In fact, they often exacerbated my condition with their examinations and tests.

"Before seeing this therapist, I had just weathered a trying, stressful three years, which started with a right-shoulder injury sustained while gardening. It would lead me through a comedy of errors, a maze of physical therapists, doctors, acupuncturists, herbalists, and new injuries, which left me with a left shoulder in worse shape than my initial right-shoulder injury. My faith in the practice of medicine was shaken, but full recovery seemed in sight, or so I thought. Thankfully, my optimism and joy for life were still intact. I knew I had enough discipline to see myself through.

"Yet this unfolding nightmare was too much to bear. My dreams of full recovery were destroyed. What now? Life was dreadfully compromised. Through trial and error I was to discover just how functionally disabled I was. I could not do simple household tasks. Could not carry three pounds. Could not turn on the kitchen faucet because the lever had too much resistance. Could not walk comfortably for more than a block. Could not ride comfortably in a car because bumps in the road would aggravate my pains. Unplugging a hairdryer from a socket would set off intense nerve pain in the neck and head. Leaning forward or backward too much in a seated position would start up the burning chest and throat pain. Couldn't sleep comfortably or continuously. The deterioration in my physical appearance was another reminder of just how bad things were getting. Who could fix this? How would I heal? Who could I trust? I was utterly frustrated, disillusioned, depressed, helpless, and hopeless.

"Then the miracle of Dr. Sha happened. I was drawn to a Whole Life Expo brochure featuring the world-renowned healer. What appealed to me was the more holistic view of the body and the less invasive diagnostic and healing process based on my rudimentary knowledge of traditional Chinese medicine and qigong. Amazingly, within two sessions, Dr. Sha's healing energy techniques would provide my first relief from the debilitating pain and restore a sense of well-being. After the first session, while the energy in my body was realigning and unblocking, it seemed as though my body was feeling every single pain it had ever experienced, all at once. It felt as if I went to the great abyss and back, but Dr. Sha assured me that was often a normal reaction. Sure enough, the pain was lifted and kept at bay.

"Without the sapping, debilitating pain, I was able to draw on my belief in myself again. I was still vulnerable, but hopeful again. Recovery was not only back in the picture, the self-healing techniques I would learn from Dr. Sha became an enjoyable and spiritually uplifting part of my day. Slowly at first, but assuredly and then dramatically, I would regain strength and feel myself healing. Needless to say, I was relieved about not having to figure out which doctor to see next. I enjoyed being able to concentrate my time and energies on self-healing. The exercises seemed effortless, like play, in contrast to the rehabilitative exercises I did before. This helped me immensely in nursing my emotional self back to a strong and healthy condition. The sparkle was back.

"I especially like how these self-healing techniques are simple, but allow for imagination and creativity. Playfulness would creep into practice because of the sweet-talking to one's body that Dr. Sha encourages. Relaxing the body, holding the various body and hand positions, along with the combination of visualizations (light, glowing health, cleansing ocean, beautiful horses) and chants (beautiful mantras or my own inventions) kept me mentally and physically engaged. But just as important, a spiritual connection forms. There is a feeling of peace and excitement all at the same time, ephemeral, but real and empowering, much like love. It was like a small private party every night, gently and powerfully moving and building energy for the restoration of health.

"Slyly, Dr. Sha's self-healing techniques heal on all planes. He emphasizes goodness and virtue, which suits my philosophy of life perfectly. With a healthy body and healthy outlook and spirit, the emotions seem to fall into place naturally, and the mind is free to dream. Mine focused on my next big trip, the ideal job, and some good chocolate. My body, mind, and spirit can't thank Dr. Sha and Heaven enough for this wonderful, joyful journey of recovery."

Although the self-healing power techniques can relieve some pain-related conditions instantly, other conditions will require days, if not weeks or months, of diligent effort. But that effort will pay off.

Melanie says: "I met Dr. Sha during a difficult time in my life. By the age of seventeen, I had undergone five surgeries for retinal detachment in my right eye and subsequently lost the vision in that eye. Now, I was facing the possibility of having a retinal detachment in my left eye. My immune system was poor. I was grossly underweight and completely miserable. The fear of going completely blind in less than a year was almost too unbearable to live with.

"I began to practice the Zhi Neng medicine healing techniques. To relieve my chronic eye pain and deal with the fear of losing my eyesight, I employed the four power-healing systems.

The mind power technique was to creatively visualize a bright spinning ball of light coming into my eyes. The sound power and soul power techniques were to continuously repeat positive messages, both silently and out loud. The body power technique was the One Hand Near, One Hand Far Method during standing-style *Dong Yi Gong*.

"During my daily activities, I would be singing to myself 'I love my eyes and my eyes love me. I can see clearly. I have perfect vision.' My family had their doubts when they saw me standing in the living room with my arms in the air chanting the natural sound of the number 1, 'ee, ee, ee, ee.' They laughed a lot but were glad that I was able to try something to help my health.

"These simple techniques really changed my life. I was happier, liked myself more, and at last had some hope. Most important, the four power-healing systems gave me the strength and knowledge I needed to heal myself.

"It worked! I am happy to report that now, four years later, my eyes are great. I have visual stability and my retinas are healthy. I've not had to undergo any further eye surgery and have even noticed vision returning in my right eye.

"I am now working as a rehabilitation assistant in various health-care facilities. The residents of these facilities need rehabilitative services for severe debilitating conditions. I help provide physiotherapy for the frail elderly. I am pleased to say that everyone I work with benefits in some way from Zhi Neng medicine and the four power-healing systems. I can give my patients hope, positive energy, and emotional support during the rehabilitation process. I feel that power healing is a wonderful complement to the existing health-care system. To me, power healing allows people to experience a more complete healing process by addressing all the integral aspects of self-healing.

"I thank Dr. Sha for his contributions to power healing and I hope that you will all enjoy its benefits as much as I have. I wish you all good luck, health, and happiness."

It took Melanie five months to completely alleviate her pain, along with the condition that caused it. But she stuck with it.

That's not always easy to do when pain is involved, so you may need to involve others and have them step in when you can't cope. This is exactly what Sabita did. When her migraines got so intense that she couldn't even concentrate on the self-healing practices she'd learned to get rid of the pain, she had her husband, Robert, to do the healing for her.

"Robert used the One Hand Near, One Hand Far Method while visualizing healing light flowing from my head to my lower abdomen to put an end to the headache within minutes," Sabita recalls. "I was always able to fall asleep without pain or medication after Robert used this specific power-healing technique."

You can even use these techniques to control externally induced pain.

"In 1997 I was diagnosed with thyroid cancer, in 1998 with gastric lymphoma, and then in 2000 with lymphoma of the spleen," says Judith. "I have endured nine rounds of chemotherapy and many painful tests, including the dreaded bone-marrow test. In fact my last bone-marrow test was so excruciatingly painful that I couldn't walk for three days afterwards. When I heard those dreaded words from my oncologist recommending I have another bone-marrow test, I went into shock and deep despair. How could I go through it again?

"I had been working with Dr. Sha and his cancer recovery group. One power-healing tool we were taught to use was singing a mantra called *Weng ar hong*. So when I went in for my bone-marrow test, I did deep-breathing exercises and sang the sacred mantra *Weng ar hong* before, during, and after the test. I was surprised when it all was over. I barely felt the long needle being injected deep into my hipbone. In fact, I couldn't believe it when the nurse told me I was finished. And, you know, I had almost no pain or discomfort afterwards. The same night of my test I was even well enough to attend the Thursday night cancer support group with Dr. Sha. In fact, that night we were singing, dancing, and standing on our feet a lot and it didn't seem to bother me at all. What a blessing! What a relief!"

Whatever the source—or duration—of your pain, you're probably obsessed with trying to eliminate it from your life. Having experienced my own crippling back pain, I understand all too well. So I urge you to find relief through the power self-healing methods. I know that suffering has sapped your energy, as well as your motivation. But you need to reclaim your life, and these techniques can help you do that, just like they helped Gaby.

"In 1986 I was busy helping an injured friend of mine on a fund-raising project as well as doing my regular job managing my husband's office," she writes. "Life was good. We had just gotten married and I felt I was on top of the world. Then, seemingly out of nowhere, one of my legs began to ache in the calf. The ache became worse and worse and progressed to the other leg. By the end of the project, I was having a difficult time standing for any length of time and I was dragging my legs around. I went to my doctor. After a number of tests and a few MRIs, I was diagnosed with multiple sclerosis.

"Needless to say, this hit me like a ton of bricks. In retrospect there had been other symptoms. Unexplained, overwhelming fatigue that would last for hours, a heavy feeling in my legs, as if I was walking through snow or water. I had attributed this simply to the aging process, as I was forty-three at the time.

"After receiving the diagnosis, my husband and I consulted with specialists all over the country. They all came back with the same diagnosis: an 'unusual' presentation of multiple sclerosis. In March 1987 I had a spinal tap. Diagnosis confirmed again: MS.

"For the next twelve years I went down many roads to try to rid my body of this dread disease. My husband was incredible through all of this. He was constantly seeking the best in medical care and advice. One thing that I think was helpful to me throughout is that I never said I 'had' MS. I said I was 'diagnosed' with MS. To me there was a difference. I did not own it. I did not take it into my being. During this time there were weeks of intense pain and times when my gait was very irregular. The pain progressed to my arms and hands. When it was very severe I went to the hospital for a shot of Demerol, which gave a few days relief. Twice I was put on a course of Prednisone. My doctors would try various medications for spasticity and pain. The symptoms would always wax and wane.

"I also tried numerous complementary and alternative approaches, including homeopathy, chiropractic, cranial-sacral work, Feldenkrais, Tibetan bowls ringing on my back, biofeedback, and acupuncture. I could go on and on. I'm not a flake or a nut, but when you experience the level of pain I was having, anything seemed worth a try, and there were times I thought I would do anything to end the pain. The saving grace was that for the periods between these bouts of pain I was able to live my life quite comfortably. Then in May 1998 I had an episode of pain that did not let up. The level of intensity grew and grew. My legs and my arms felt like they were going to explode. After the shots of Demerol, I was put on Tegretol and Neurontin. Both medications are used to control seizures. This only reduced the pain somewhat. In addition, I was given more painkillers, Vicodin, then Lortab.

"We were searching frantically for a solution. Suddenly, there was a major change in direction. A reexamination by the medical director of an MS center resulted in his saying after fourteen years: 'I do not know what you have. It is serious, but it is not MS.' At the same time, a wonderful neurologist whom a friend of mine found offered to study my charts. He recommended that I obtain metabolic studies. So I had spinal fluid drawn and sent to one of the few places in the country where they do these kinds of studies. The findings were extraordinary. The level of one of my enzymes, S-adenosylhomosysteine or SAH, was between sixteen and twenty times normal! They had never seen such high levels. To be sure, they sent my spinal fluid to the U. S. Department of Toxicology laboratory in Arkansas. They confirmed the finding.

"To me, this was wonderful news. I finally had an explanation for the extreme pain. I learned that SAH affects the neurotransmitters, which in turn affect the pain pathways. However, I was still in extreme pain, and something worse had happened. Not only were my central and peripheral nervous systems being affected; now my sympathetic nervous system had become involved. I began experiencing extreme nausea and vomiting. I had no appetite and went from 118 pounds to 99 pounds. I was hospitalized in January 1999 and put on intravenous feeding and strong painkillers. The prognosis was poor. Though he did not tell me at the time, a doctor friend of my husband told him that sometimes they are not able to turn these things around. A certain percentage of the patients do not survive.

"The biochemist who analyzed my spinal fluid suggested I try SAM-e, which is an enzyme that works synergistically with SAH. As they had never seen anybody with my condition, they were trying something that had no history, just hoping it would work. I was released from the hospital with a prescription for SAM-e, and methadone for pain. I was still nauseous and had no appetite. My weight was continuing to go down. I felt as though I was beginning to know death personally. It was very frightening, knowing I had to eat in order to survive, but not being able to. As I sit here today, it does not make sense. Just put the food in your mouth and swallow! But I couldn't, and only now do I understand that it really was not possible. I have since spoken with people who have had the same experience, so I know it is a real physiological problem, not a psychological one. I went down to 89 pounds. My digestive system was shutting down. Surviving became my total focus.

"I thank God for my friends through all of this. It is because of them that I can tell this story today. They monitored my intake of food and supplements daily and referred me to a man who offered to help me. This man did some energy work on my stomach. I could feel the heat through his hands, and I heard my stomach growl and snarl. At the end of the session he picked some lettuce from his garden, handed it to me, and said, 'You heard those noises, that was your stomach waking up. Now go home and eat!' I was not able to eat lettuce, but I was able to eat a little rice, and bit by bit as I worked with the nutritionist and had body and energy work done, my appetite returned. My oldest friend from the first grade flew three thousand miles to stay with me for a week and cook and feed me. I was so nurtured!

"So then it was no longer that my life was fragile, but I was still experiencing pain between 50 and 80 percent of the time. I was able to keep it bearable with the methadone, but the quality of my life certainly was compromised. Then late last year I began to attend a healing program run by Drs. Sha and Gray. It was a three-month cancer group study in which we would learn to heal one another and ourselves. This has turned my health around.

"Initially, I went to the program to support my friend who had been diagnosed with lung cancer. What I have learned in the six months since has been incredible for the quality of my life. When I began with the group, I was experiencing pain between 50 to 80 percent of the time and was emotionally sad and exhausted from being in so much pain. Using the scale that doctors like so much these days, on a scale of one to ten the pain was often around five or six (at least no longer what it was—level fourteen—when I was in the hospital). Still, every night I would awaken with a strong burning pain in the soles of my feet, lasting for an hour or more.

"Dr. Sha introduced me to his power self-healing program. This is not a mystery. We all have the ability to understand and absorb this teaching. When people are very ill, they are open to help, open to the miracle of life, and perhaps better able to feel a certain proximity to God, especially with the help of Dr. Sha, who has studied many years with Buddhist masters. Although he is a very verbal and demonstrative master, Dr. Sha was able to affect me on a cellular level. There has been a shift in my being. The most wonderful thing has been the reduction of the pain. I received and continue to receive valuable tools that have helped. First of all I chant. Now, my chanting is not regular. I don't have a certain time of day that I do it, although I tell myself that when the garden is finished and my little meditation corner is set, I will. However, I find myself chanting silently very often throughout the day. Sometimes I awaken from sleep chanting. The pain in the bottom of my feet comes only occasionally and at a very low level. It goes away when I put the soles of my feet together and chant or if I move the energy away from my feet with visualizations of light flowing up from my feet to my lower abdomen. The leg pain that used to be almost constant is now rare.

"It frightens me a bit to say how much the power self-healing techniques have helped me. It's almost too good to be true. Yet it's too good not to say it. It's too good not to pass it on and share with others, especially those who are suffering as I suffered."

It takes commitment and a true desire and willingness to learn these techniques and then apply those that seem to fit you best.

But in many instances, only by giving your body a break from the pain can it relearn to be pain free. Ironically, chronic pain can be like a bad habit. Just as a person can get so used to having painful relationships that they become the norm, your body can become accustomed to experiencing pain—however negative that is. By giving your body a reprieve from that pain, breaking up the energy blockages, and promoting the flow of *chi,* your body will heal itself.

BEYOND THE BODY

As we all know, pain is not only physical. Ironically, Americans seem to suffer more than most from emotional challenges ranging from dissatisfaction to depression (the latter of which Andrew Weil says is "now epidemic in our culture"[1]). In this country, one out of four women, one out of ten men, and one out of twenty adolescents will experience depression.[2]

Of course, there's a direct correlation between emotional and physical health. Roger Jahnke, in *The Healer Within,* writes:

The scientific research on the effect of emotions on health can be stated simply. Body chemistry shifts and literally produces poisons when a person is in a sustained state of anger, fear, grief, frustration, or worry. Physiologically, when a person is in a stress state, the overactivity of the nervous system taxes the adrenal gland. This creates a lack of responsiveness in the body's self-healing capacity. The immune cells are unable to get clear direction when the adrenal is overactive or deficient, leading to the risk of cancer and other immune deficiency disorders. And stress builds tension in the circulatory system, elevating the risk of heart attack or stroke.

These findings have been reconfirmed in hundreds of studies. It has also been clearly established that sustained joy, contentment, and security cause a shift in the body chemistry to produce healing elixirs.[3]

I would probably explain things a little differently and say that factors such as strong emotion can cause excess energy to build up in the body. For example, if you get very angry, your liver cells vibrate more strongly than usual. A high-intensity field forms around the liver, which affects other organs in the body. For instance, this excess energy may affect the stomach and cause a feeling of fullness, pain, poor appetite, or indigestion. If the anger is not released, the liver cells vibrate even more and radiate even more energy. Over time, the excess energy accumulated may produce inflammation or a tumor in the liver itself or in other organs.

Either way you look at it, however, finding your emotional balance is key to restoring and maintaining health. Conversely, getting healthy by promoting better *chi* flow and eliminating energy blockages in your body is the key to regaining or maintaining your emotional well-being. Thankfully, depression and related emotional disorders can be self-healed. Just ask Paul.

"I was seriously fatigued and burned out in my job as a counselor, as well as from dealing with two deaths in my family in two years. This resulted in a bout of depression," Paul recalls. "I was no longer functioning well at work, with my children, or in my relationships. I was very numb. During this time, I went to several doctors for my fatigue and several counselors and therapists for my depression. At the same time, our family took on another child whose mother had died. Life had become overwhelming. My response was to tune out.

"We saw our family counselor for advice about how to deal with the new child. Our counselor had been in a serious car accident and was seeing Dr. Sha for chronic pain. She told us it was working for her and recommended that I see Dr. Sha for my problems.

"I was very suspicious at first. I had tried counseling, antidepressants, and therapy. Nothing really helped. I was still fatigued and depressed. I was also beginning to suffer from panic attacks. Because I was getting desperate, I decided to check Dr. Sha out.

"My wife and I went to one of Dr. Sha's presentations. At first, I thought what he was doing was all kind of nuts. But for some reason I found myself going to see Dr. Sha a few months later, after taking a stress leave from work.

"I decided to try it. Within a month, my depression started to lift. My energy started to come back. Although I was broke, I decided to buy some of Dr. Sha's audiotapes and began to practice. I tried the golden healing ball, the numbers 1 to 11, and the special healing number mantra 3396815. I also started to practice a number of his self-healing exercises. These have worked much better than any antidepressants I've ever taken—and with no side effects!

"I practice almost every day. I do the exercises and say the numbers like a daily mantra each time I go for a walk, or whenever I think about it. My anxiety is gone. I'm feeling better and I'm not only going back to work rested, but with confidence and energy."

RESTORING EMOTIONAL BALANCE

In my study of the conditions of depression, anxiety, worry, sadness, and fear, I have found that these emotional problems are related to the health of different organs and can actually be the cause of sickness in the organs. A person with an open Third Eye can see when an unhealthy person has an emotional disorder. The emotional condition will turn up as darkness in the Message Center. The more severe the emotional disorder, the darker the Message Center.

If you're depressed, anxious, sad, or fearful because of family relationships, work, stress, physical illness, or anything else in your life that bothers you, I want you to try the following exercises.

For each one, start with basic relaxation techniques. Give yourself a few minutes to relax from head to toe; relax from skin to organs to bones; let your body completely relax; let every cell relax as much as you can.

Why must you relax the body and the cells? When you completely relax, your cells will be able to expand and contract freely. Your cells will breathe in and breathe out, expand and contract, better. Imagine that you have stress and tension in your neck. Your neck feels stiff. Your head feels heavy because the cells in your neck and head are contracting more than they are expanding. Energy is blocked in the area of stress. When you completely relax your body, the cells breathe freely, vibrate freely, and expand and contract in a more balanced way.

DEPRESSION

In the exercise for depression, you will be using your mind to concentrate on your chest. While you are completely relaxed, you will be focusing on your Message Center (2½ *cun* behind the midpoint between your nipples) and visualizing bright white light radiating from inside your chest in this area, which is also known as the heart chakra.

This exercise will help you work on improving the quality of the messages received in your Message Center. After as short a period as one week, you will notice how much your emotional disorder has improved. When you open your Third Eye, you will be able to see your Message Center becoming lighter and lighter. Even without opening your Third Eye, you will notice your depression is improving. It may, however, take you a few days, weeks, or months to recover completely from your emotional disorder.

Healing Practice
Prepare (Body Power Technique)

Take any comfortable position (standing, sitting, or lying down). Relax completely. Locate and focus on your Message Center.

Chant (Sound Power Technique)

Tell your Message Center: "I love my Message Center. I love my Message Center. I love my Message Center. I love my Message Center. Please expand and contract, expand and contract. Please expand and contract, expand and contract. Please expand and contract, expand and contract. Please expand and contract, expand and contract.

"Message Center vibrating, Message Center vibrating, Message Center vibrating, Message Center vibrating . . ."

Visualize (Mind Power Technique)

Visualize bright white light radiating in your Message Center. "Light, light, light, light . . ." Put purity into your Message Center. Think love, care, compassion, sincerity, honesty, integrity in your Message Center.

Communicate (Soul Power Technique)

"I forgive myself. I forgive others. Purity, purity, purity, purity. Peace, peace, peace, peace. Love, love, love, love . . ."

Close (Soul Power Technique)

Say "*Hao, hao, hao.* Thank you, thank you, thank you."

Practice Time

Spend a minimum of fifteen minutes doing this exercise, two or three times a day.

When asked to describe her biggest stumbling block, the one that has often shaped her decisions and her actions, Sharon can sum it up in a single word: fear. "Fear of who I am, fear of where I am going, fear of how I look, fear of relationships, fear of beauty, fear of moving, fear of career," she explains. "The list goes on." By using message and energy techniques like the one above, "I am in tune and then gain and have that confidence to manifest my next move."

Figuring out what it takes to self-heal emotionally can make a huge difference not only in your health, but also in the overall quality of your life. Just ask someone like Dr. Peter Hudoba, an internationally acclaimed neurosurgeon, researcher, and university department head, who has had to battle that syndrome known as "burnout."

"As a neurosurgeon, I have always been excited by the brain, and not just the anatomy, but also the power of the mind behind the brain, says Dr. Hudoba." "One slip of my hand during any part of an eight-hour or longer surgery on someone's brain to remove a tumor can result in instant paralysis, or death for that matter. My hands have to remain steady and precise for hours and hours. So to balance out my heavily technical and excruciatingly detail-oriented profession, I've found peace and solace in the pursuit of higher states of consciousness. Exploring the inner dimensions of my own mind has been quite powerful. In fact I have been studying Taoism for twenty years. The ultimate goal of Taoism is enlightenment and opening of consciousness. And the ability to use these skills to do better, more precise surgery and simply to steady my hands has been life-saving. The basic skills of meditation practiced daily over these years have greatly helped my concentration. That is perhaps why I am such a sought-after brain surgeon.

"I went into medicine to heal and help people at a time when they desperately needed help. To save lives, give hope, and restore faith is indeed a distinct honor and a privilege. The amazing part of my job is the closeness I experience every day to the life force of a human being. Over the years medicine has become less patient-centered and more mechanical and systematized. Many times I have to struggle to keep my healing spirit alive. Without that innate healing spirit, I lose my ability to instinctively know what is wrong with my patients

"One of the ways I have found to keep my intuition and instincts alive is to attend spiritual-growth seminars and lectures. But that hasn't always been enough.

"After one particularly rough month of hospital red tape and some messy politics, I decided I really needed a break. My spirits were dashed, and some days I even felt like quitting. I needed to find the right workshop or lecture. I began searching and learned of a program with Dr. Sha. In one weekend I learned a powerful chant, *Weng ar hong,* some soul power techniques and soul communication techniques. Through guided imagery and soul work and prayer, my ability to focus returned.

"I had been trained in very advanced meditation techniques, which I practiced daily for twenty years. In all my twenty years of practicing Taoism, I never had such a powerful experience. I was brought into such a state of peace and divine awareness that I felt deeply transformed. Such divine peace and awareness. I was happy for the first time in years. And in that state of happiness I saw how unhappy I had been.

"I returned to work a different person. Many of the other doctors noticed the visible difference in me. Many said my face seemed to glow. Some said I looked remarkably different, like I had lost weight or something. Everyone said I looked so happy and rested. My family was the most amazed at the change. I just had to laugh.

"The greatest benefit came when I was back in surgery standing on my feet for another eight- to ten-hour life-threatening operation and I chanted the *Weng ar hong* mantra in my head. The sound power technique and the mind power technique steadied my hands, and before I knew it the operation was completed perfectly. Absolutely perfectly. I will always be grateful for my healing hands and these powerful techniques.

"Now I enjoy my home life more as well. And I am sure my wife and family and even my black Labrador retriever like having me around now too."

Anger

In traditional Chinese medicine, all emotional problems are related to internal organs. If you have an emotional problem, it will affect your organs' health and vice versa. For example, if you get upset or angry, it will affect the health of your liver. Conversely, if your liver is unhealthy, you will easily get angry and upset. But five special healing sounds can vibrate all your major internal organs, body tissues, and emotions. As I show you how, don't hesitate to try these out for yourself.

To self-heal emotional anger and upset, you will be chanting the special healing sound *jiao* (pronounced "jow") to vibrate the liver (which is connected to those emotions) to promote the liver's energy flow, to remove energy blockages in the liver, and to self-heal the liver. As the liver's condition improves, anger and upset will release and disappear.

Healing Practice
Prepare (Body Power Technique)

Sit, stand, or lie down comfortably and relax completely.

Chant (Sound Power Technique)

Say "*Jiao* (pronounced 'jow'), *jiao, jiao, jiao . . .* " Chant for at least five minutes, the longer the better.

Visualize (Mind Power Technique)

As you chant *jiao*, at the same time visualize bright green light radiating in your liver area (located inside the lower right ribs on the side). Visualize the green light getting brighter and brighter while chanting: "Healthy liver cells, healthy liver cells, healthy liver cells, healthy liver cells. Peaceful liver cells, peaceful liver cells, peaceful liver cells, peaceful liver cells."

Communicate (Soul Power Technique)

Communicate directly with your liver. "I love my liver, I love my liver, I love my liver, I love my liver. I love my liver *hun* (the soul of the liver, pronounced 'huen'). I love my liver *hun*. I love my liver *hun*. I love my liver *hun*. Liver cells vibrating, liver cells vibrating, liver cells vibrating, liver cells vibrating.

"*Jiao, jiao, jiao, jiao.* Perfect liver, perfect liver, perfect liver, perfect liver. Happy liver cells, happy liver cells, happy liver cells, happy liver cells. Dancing liver cells, dancing liver cells, dancing liver cells, dancing liver cells. Intelligent liver cells, intelligent liver cells, intelligent liver cells, intelligent liver cells. Happy DNA and RNA inside liver cells, happy DNA and RNA inside liver cells, happy DNA and RNA inside liver cells, happy DNA and RNA inside liver cells. Purify liver cells, purify liver cells, purify liver cells, purify liver cells. Balance transformation between the matter inside the liver cells and the energy outside the liver cells. Balance transformation between the matter inside the liver cells and the energy outside the liver cells. Balance transformation between the matter inside the liver cells and the energy outside the liver cells. Balance transformation between the matter inside the liver cells and the energy outside the liver cells."

Close (Soul Power Technique)

Say "*Hao, hao, hao.* Thank you, thank you, thank you."

Practice Time

Continue for at least five minutes, the longer the better. Practice this three to five times a day.

ANXIETY

When you can't stop worrying about something, you can correct that by chanting the special healing sound *gong* (pronounced "gohng") to vibrate the spleen, promote the spleen's energy flow, remove energy blockages in the spleen, and self-heal the spleen. As the spleen's condition improves, excessive worry will release and disappear, along with a handful of related physical conditions. According to traditional Chinese medicine, the spleen is in charge of digestion and absorption. When you are worried, it affects your spleen's health, which in turn causes poor digestion, indigestion, poor absorption, gas, and other symptoms in the digestive system. Conversely, if you have spleen problems, you are prone to get overly worried.

Healing Practice
Prepare (Body Power Technique)

Use any comfortable position (sitting, standing, or lying down). Relax your body.

Chant (Sound Power Technique)

"*Gong* (pronounced 'gohng'), *gong, gong, gong* . . ." Chant continuously.

Visualize (Mind Power Technique)

While you are chanting, visualize bright yellow light radiating in the spleen area (located inside the lower left ribs on the side).

Communicate (Soul Power Technique)

"Spleen cells vibrating, spleen cells vibrating, spleen cells vibrating, spleen cells vibrating. I love my spleen *yi* (the soul of the spleen, pronounced 'yee'), I love my spleen *yi*, I love my spleen *yi*, I love my spleen *yi*. Spleen cells functioning better, spleen cells functioning better, spleen cells functioning better, spleen cells functioning better. Bright yellow light radiating in the spleen, bright yellow light radiating in the spleen, bright yellow light radiating in the spleen, bright yellow light radiating in the spleen. Good emotions, good emotions, good emotions, good emotions. *Gong, gong, gong, gong . . .*"

Close (Soul Power Technique)

Say "*Hao, hao, hao.* Thank you, thank you, thank you."

Practice Time

Continue to chant *gong* for at least five minutes, the longer the better. Practice this three to five times a day.

SADNESS AND GRIEF

Emotional sadness and grief can be alleviated by stimulating cellular vibration in the lungs, since the lungs are so strongly related to sadness and grief. You may have noticed that when you are sad and grieving, you're more likely have lung conditions, such as shortness of breath and a resulting lack of energy. Conversely, if you have lung problems, you will more easily become sad and grieving. Chanting *shang* (pronounced "shahng") will vibrate the lung cells, promote the lungs' energy flow, remove energy blockages, and self-heal lung conditions as well as emotional sadness and grief.

Healing Practice
Prepare (Body Power Technique)

Take any comfortable position (standing, sitting, or lying down) and relax.

Chant (Sound Power Technique)

"Shang (pronounced "shahng"), *shang, shang, shang . . ."* Chant continuously.

Visualize (Mind Power Technique)

While you are chanting, visualize bright white light radiating in the lungs. Chant as fast as you can and visualize as bright a white light as you can. "Light, light, light, light." Visualize the bright white light radiating in your lungs. "Light, light, light, light. Light, light, light, light."

Communicate (Soul Power Technique)

"Clear lungs, clear lungs, clear lungs, clear lungs. I love my lung *po* (the soul of the lungs, pronounced 'poe'). I request my lung *po* to balance the transformation between the matter inside my lungs and the energy outside my lungs. I love every cell of my lungs. I enjoy my lung cells. I appreciate my lung cells. *Shang, shang, shang, shang . . ."*

Close (Soul Power Technique)

Say "*Hao, hao, hao.* Thank you, thank you, thank you."

Practice Time

Continue for at least five minutes, the longer the better. Practice this three to five times a day.

FEAR

You can get a handle on fear and fright by chanting the special healing sound *yu* (pronounced "yih") to vibrate the kidneys, promoting the kidneys' energy flow, removing energy blockages in the kidneys, and self-healing the kidneys. As the kidneys' condition improves, fear and fright will release and disappear. In addition, your propensity to feel fearful will diminish as well.

Healing Practice
Prepare (Body Power Technique)

Use any comfortable position (sitting, standing, or lying down) and relax completely.

Chant (Sound Power Technique)

Chant "*Yu* (pronounced 'yih'), *yu, yu, yu . . .* " continuously.

Visualize (Mind Power Technique)

While you are chanting, visualize bright blue light radiating in the kidney area (located in the back just above the waist on either side of the spine).

Communicate (Soul Power Technique)

Communicate with your kidneys: "I love my kidneys, I love my kidneys, I love my kidneys, I love my kidneys. Kidney cells vibrating, kidney cells vibrating, kidney cells vibrating, kidney cells vibrating. Happy kidney cells, happy kidney cells, happy kidney cells, happy kidney cells. I love my kidney *zhi* (the soul of the kidneys, pronounced 'djih'), I love my kidney *zhi*, I love my kidney *zhi*, I love my kidney *zhi*. I request my kidney *zhi* to help my kidneys recover and to take out fear and fright."

Close (Soul Power Technique)

Say "*Hao, hao, hao.* Thank you, thank you, thank you."

Practice Time

Continue for at least five minutes, the longer the better. Practice this three to five times a day.

OVEREXCITEMENT

Ironically, any excessive emotion, even if it's positive, can get you into trouble. When overexcitement or too much happiness come into play, chant the special healing sound *zhi* (pronounced "djih") to vibrate the heart, promote the heart's energy flow, remove energy blockages in the heart, and self-heal the heart. As the heart's condition improves, overexcited and overhappy emotions will release and disappear.

Why does this work? The heart is related to happiness and joy. If you are overly happy or overjoyed, those intense emotions will gradually create an unhealthy condition in your heart. Too much laughter can even become a problem. Though the link between laughter and healing has been well established, you probably know from experience that if you laugh too much, you'll wind up feeling tired and weak. That's because too much laughter makes the heart cells overexpand before they contract. Cellular vibration becomes unbalanced and the cells feel tired, causing the person to feel tired. For those with heart problems, overstimulation or overexcitement may bring on a heart attack. Conversely, if a person has a heart problem, that person will tend to get excited easily and be more sensitive to excitement.

The following exercise will bring both emotions and heart back into balance.

Healing Practice
Prepare (Body Power Technique)

Take any comfortable position (sitting, standing, or lying down). Relax.

Chant (Sound Power Technique)

Chant *"Zhi* (pronounced 'djih'), *zhi, zhi, zhi . . ."* continuously.

Visualize (Mind Power Technique)

At the same time, visualize a bright red light radiating in your heart area.

Communicate (Soul Power Technique)

Communicate with your heart: "I love my heart. I love my heart *shen* (the soul of the heart, pronounced 'shehn'). Heart cells vibrating, heart cells vibrating, heart cells vibrating, heart cells vibrating. I care for my heart cells, I care for my heart cells, I care for my heart cells, I care for my heart cells. Improve the quality of my heart cells, improve the quality of my heart cells, improve the quality of my heart cells, improve the quality of my heart cells. Heart blood circulates better, heart blood circulates better, heart blood circulates better, heart blood circulates better. Kind heart, kind heart, kind heart, kind heart.

"Peaceful heart, peaceful heart, peaceful heart, peaceful heart. Enlighten my heart, enlighten my heart, enlighten my heart, enlighten my heart. Perfect heart, perfect heart, perfect heart, perfect heart.

"Good emotions, good emotions, good emotions, good emotions. Balanced emotions, balanced emotions, balanced emotions, balanced emotions."

Close (Soul Power Technique)

Say "*Hao, hao, hao.* Thank you, thank you, thank you."

Practice Time

Continue to chant and visualize for at least five minutes, the longer the better. Practice this three to five times a day.

Though the relationship between your organs and emotions is a close one, it may take time for the physical symptoms to appear. Of course, by being attuned to your feelings and using these self-healing techniques to deal with them, you may be able to avoid the physical fallout entirely. Your self-healing efforts on this front may also prove to be just what the doctor ordered when it comes to handling your personal—and even business—affairs. That's certainly what Mark found.

"I am the vice president and general manager of a major auto dealership," Mark writes. "I am responsible for over 150 employees, as well as for the overall performance and success of the dealership. We have been the number one retail dealership in our region for the past eight years and one of the top fifty dealerships in the United States. This business demands a great deal of an individual. We are open seven days a weak, twelve to sixteen hours a day. We face daily pressures from the manufacturer to perform, and our customers expect complete satisfaction.

"I first heard Dr. Sha on the radio one morning while driving to work. As a prostate cancer survivor, I was overwhelmed with the positive approaches that Dr. Sha was discussing. I felt that Dr. Sha could provide me with positive methods of self-healing that not only would prevent any cancer recurrence, but also continue to improve my overall health, as well strengthen my spiritual beliefs and powers.

"I then attended two group meetings with Dr. Sha and began working with him one on one. Since then I have seen significant improvements in my health, my attitude, and my temperament. He has improved my total overall well-being by helping me achieve a newfound calmness and total positive outlook toward any problem or situation. In addition, he has created release mechanisms within my body to defuse anger and negativity.

"I have also found that my interpersonal skills have improved when dealing with my employees, whether it is a business matter or a personal matter that is affecting their work performance. This too I ascribe to Dr. Sha and his power self-healing methods.

"The business world is filled with pressure and high expectations. These demands can shorten one's life or career. I consider it a blessing that God has delivered to me my relationship with Dr. Sha. I have the results to prove his value to me now and in the future. Dr. Sha has given me the confidence to continue to excel and to be the best that I can be as a husband, father, citizen, athlete, and business leader."

Of course, certain emotions—and conditions—are harder to control than others. But even those, once managed, offer unexpected opportunity.

14

FROM PATIENT TO HEALER

There's nothing quite like the emotional impact of being told that you have cancer—the big "C." Sadly, the feelings of fear and despair that so often accompany the diagnosis can be as detrimental as the cancer itself.

"A year ago, at the age of fifty-six, I was diagnosed for the first time with stage-two breast cancer," says Kay. "With a masters in social work, I have worked for the last eight years with people with life-threatening illnesses, mental illnesses, and other life crises. My experience with these conditions didn't stave off any of the normal human reactions when I myself was diagnosed with cancer. I lost my balance and my center. I felt like I was tossing and turning in a world where no one had any answers and yet I was being forced to make choices between equally jarring alternatives.

"Along with fear and confusion, I felt helpless and powerless. My doctors themselves often disagreed with each other's recommendations. I felt like I was pulled into a giant machine that worked on my body without fully understanding my body, much less the mind and spirit that inhabited it and influenced it so profoundly."

Helping people to regain their quality of life has fueled all of my self-healing teachings. Nowhere is that challenge greater than with those diagnosed with incurable diseases, and most especially with cancer. So in the fall of 2000, John Gray and I started the Cancer Recovery Pilot Program to see whether our efforts and self-healing methods could really make a difference. After three months, the intended duration of the program, the progress we saw made us decide to continue the program indefinitely. But Kay's words speak to the program's impact more directly than I ever could.

"It wasn't until I became a part of the Cancer Recovery Pilot Program with Drs. Sha and Gray that I began to expand the possibilities of dealing with my illness. This program offered a more integrated approach—at the body, mind, and soul levels. At last I found someone who didn't view my body mechanistically, but who addressed my cancer condition in a more holistic way. In Dr. Sha, I found a master teacher who was not only trained as a medical doctor, but who also was a master of the processes of the mind, body, and soul. At last I felt that my entire being was brought into the healing arena. My scattered mind and energies began to focus. My confusion and fears were quieted.

"In addition to having my condition addressed in a holistic way, I was also moved by the sense of empowerment in the underlying focus on self-healing. Although we needed the mastery of Dr. Sha for many things, he was also teaching us to take care of ourselves, showing us practical ways to use sound, movement, visualization, energy, and the support of the divine to accelerate the course of our healing.

"One of the teachings that affected me deeply was the whole concept of communicating with our souls, with the souls of each of our organs, with the souls of our very cells. I also liked working with various hand positions to affect energy flow. This was a key for me. I had never related to my body in a very personal way; even anatomy classes were kind of distant. But over time, I began to form an intimate connection with my body—with its extraordinary complexity and mystery, its strength and delicacy, its wisdom and responsiveness—and its capacity to heal. This energized and motivated my commitment to healing work. Now when I turn to my body, I feel a lot of gratitude and intimacy.

"The work also energized and enlivened my spirit. Working with a group of people facing life-threatening illness and having the shared intention of supporting the healing of each other as well as our own was powerful unto itself. Working with the guidance of a master teacher like Dr. Sha, whose boundless energy, commitment, and sincerity are apparent in everything he does, added even greater spirit to our work together. And finally, invoking the blessing of our Heaven Team, as Dr. Sha refers to our helper deities, expanded the arena of healing to greater dimensions. There were times when I barely had an ounce of energy to drag myself to our meetings—but by the time I left, my fatigue vanished and I felt alive, energized, and physically regenerated. I believe this matter of the spirit is very important for cancer recovery."

THE FORMATION OF CANCER CELLS

In traditional Chinese medicine, there is a very famous statement: *"Chi ju ze cheng xing. Chi shan ze cheng feng."* Translation: "Accumulation of vital energy *(chi)* may cause a growth (a benign tumor or cancer). Dissipation of the vital energy *(chi)* will reduce or eliminate the growth, just like the wind flows away." This important theory in traditional Chinese medicine, established five thousand years ago, continues to guide clinical practice for treating tumors and cancer.

According to Zhi Neng medicine theory, there are two ways cancer cells are formed. First, if any factor—emotional, environmental, genetic, etc.—causes the cells to contract more intensely and for longer periods of time than they expand, then lots of matter inside the cells transforms to energy outside the cells. This large amount of energy outside the cells accumulates in the space between the cells. Because this high-density energy cannot then flow fast enough to other parts of the body, the matter remaining inside the cells cannot properly transform to energy in the space outside the cells. Thus, the matter will accumulate inside the cells. The shapes of the cells, the membranes of the cells, the nuclei of the cells will change. The cells will first become precancerous cells and then develop into cancer cells.

Second, when a great deal of energy accumulates in the space between the cells, this highly accumulated energy will itself produce new cancer cells.

As we've seen over and over again, the solution is to dissipate those energy blockages and get the *chi* to flow properly again, thereby allowing the cells to return to normal. That's our focus in the cancer recovery program. Our goal is not only for participants to heal themselves physically and emotionally, but to support and heal others as well. Our methodology uses all the power self-healing techniques you're now familiar with. And just as I hope you will, we try and make them as much fun as possible. We sing and chant. We hold hands and dance. We learn, work, laugh, celebrate, and, when necessary, commiserate together. Despite the illness that brings the group together, we have fun.

"I came to Dr. Sha with the hope of healing an ovarian cyst enclosing a small tumor, where 'iffy' cells are fused to the surface wall," says Suzanne. "The first time I experienced his healing work, he invited all those present with cancer to take a risk and join him at the front of the room. Then he asked for a person with a backache to volunteer. He asked the people with cancer to point one hand at their cancer site and point the other hand at the volunteer's back. I thought that we cancer people would surely kill the volunteer with our bad energy. Instead, the volunteer's backache disappeared.

"Dr. Sha then introduced the notion that cancer is due to a blockage of energy in the body where excess energy has accumulated. Rather than being bad, this blocked energy—which can be understood as light—can be released to help others.

"I soon learned how to focus and visualize this blocked energy as light extending from my ovary, through my body, and on through my fingers to the area needing healing in another person. With a roomful of such focused people extending healing light, we have seen miracles over time, and even in the moment.

"I have incorporated these self-healing and healing techniques into my daily spiritual practice, an integration of West and East. I am more aware of how intimate I am with the spiritual world, a parallel world operating in my own time and space. This intimacy with spirit allows me to pray, meditate, and chant with total confidence that I am heard. This intimacy assures me that the healings I participate in are indeed a reality, a reality that I can expect when I ask for the grace of healing for others and for myself. As a result of Dr. Sha's healing methods and teachings, I have the expectation that my ovary has been healed. Much more than that, I have experienced the alleviation of a year-long depression and I have realized a more confident attitude toward myself and others, and toward life.

"Life can be stressful. I know mine is. But now I can chant 'God's light' and watch myself as I calm down, slow down, and experience the world in a new way with more clarified, focused energy. Now I can communicate and pray not just to feel better, but to truly communicate with the Great Ones. My life has changed for the better and I am able to live as a more powerful vehicle for service, to others, and to myself."

Traditional Chinese medicine explains that emotional anger is one of the main causes of cancer, because the anger causes *chi* to accumulate, which in turn causes a tumor (or cancer) to begin. Turning off that anger, whatever it stems from, and channeling that excess energy elsewhere is part of what our program is all about. We also get participants not only to accept the cancer that is now a part of them, but to love it.

Does that sound strange? Impossible? It's really not. In *Spontaneous Healing*, Andrew Weil tells the story of a Japanese cancer survivor who opted to check himself into a new healing retreat in the Japanese Alps instead of staying in the hospital. Weil quotes his friend as saying: "The clean air and water invigorated me, and I became aware of the natural healing power that was in me and around me. Gradually, I began to realize that I had created my own cancer. I had created it by my behavior. And as I came to that realization, I saw that I had to love my cancer, not attack it as an enemy. It was part of me, and I had to love my whole self."[1]

Accepting and loving your body—even in a less than perfect condition—is what gives you the power to change it. How? By telling your body what you want, and then giving it what it needs to change. "Cancer cells, you made a mistake," participants in the cancer recovery group say out loud in a strong, certain voice. "You went the wrong direction. You made a mistake. Go back the other way. You can do it. We will help." Then they chant "Cancer cells return to normal cells, cancer cells return to normal cells" as they visualize a healing light or golden ball directed at themselves or others.

"The kind of energy work that Dr. Gray and Dr. Sha do is very similar to prayer, except it is highly interactive," says Joan Kasich, whose study found such concrete improvement in the body chemistries of participants in the cancer recovery program. "It has been known for centuries how powerful prayer is. Prayer alkalizes the body. Because the energy work in the cancer recovery program is concentrated and intense, I believe it causes an alkaline-forming reaction in the body. Plus the members of the group continually serve each other by participating in each other's energy healing. Service to others creates an alkaline state. I am not talking about a 'do-gooder' mentality, but an awareness of taking care of someone who is forlorn, offering money to someone in a financial bind, helping a neighbor fix a plumbing problem, preparing wonderful food for guests, or bringing laughter to an ill friend. The energy work is a continual loop of service to self and service to others."

Whichever explanation you buy, there's no quibbling with the results. I'll let Dr. Peter Hudoba share his impressions of our group with you, as well as his analysis of its impact on participants:

"The whole atmosphere of the session was remarkable. These were not the cancer patients I know from my practice (as a neurosurgeon, I have treated many cancer patients). Despite having advanced cases of cancer, the participants were mostly enthusiastic, vibrant with the power to defeat terrible illness, and eager to enjoy what was left. I said to one of my friends, 'I see the true spirit of American pioneers—no way they would ever quit!'

"But on the energy level, it was more than that. Over the years, I developed the capability to perceive things on an energy level, to feel the moving force behind events.

"The best way to describe what I felt at that time is that it was like watching the movie *Battle of the Titans* or a war between good and evil. The whole room resonated, and I felt various energies expanding, moving, exchanging. During mantra recitations, I saw the spiritual energy coming down like a bolt of lightning on some of the participants. Participants were not the passive, receiving, unhappy beings I know from my practice; they were actively helping each other, combining all they had in unison to defeat their common adversary, participating totally in the healing process. Master Sha, like a director of big symphonic orchestra, was slowly moving between them, doing this and that, manipulating all this cacophony into one focused direction.

"It was a moving, remarkable experience that reached the deepest chords of my being. In front of me, there was concise, condensed meaning of all the spiritual teachings I have ever studied: the Bible, Vedas, yoga, *Tao Te Ching,* Buddhist sutras; it was all there in one short movie. I was directly experiencing the suffering of our human existence, the way to salvation, the savior, merciful God. If I ever have truly felt that God is, it was there!

"As if this was not enough as it was, my conceptual mind still wanted 'proper proof' of whether this was really working. Using a standardized scientific method, we studied participants' improvement in well-being by means of questionnaires and then statistically analyzed the data. We found that after three months of treatment, participants improved significantly in terms of quality of life, in emotional stability, and in cognitive functioning and had reduced pain, fatigue, insomnia, and loss of appetite. We don't know yet which type of cancer is the most susceptible to being helped by this method and what degree of recovery one can hope for. However, the results were so encouraging that we are going to continue with this study to find that out."

As welcome as such further study will be, I don't need statistics or scientific analysis to confirm how much better so many of the group's participants now feel.

"I've gotten a lot of benefits from this group—and I'm not the only one," says Susan, who joined for the initial three-month pilot study and then stayed. "This work has been very powerful.

The group energy uplifts all of us. The more people practicing in unison, the stronger the energy. And this work is energy work, moving our energy through our bodies and healing ourselves.

"I can remember walking in the first night and the first few meetings. There were a lot of people who were very ill, people who had to lie down on the benches in the church pews, not having a whole lot of energy. By the end of the first month, people were coming to the group with smiles on their faces and laughing. Everybody was feeling better.

"That's certainly been so true for me. Before the group, my core—my spiritual core—was not nearly as happy as it is today. The group has given me a lot of self-confidence. It's given me a lot of joy. And it's given me back my health.

"When I started, I had a spot in my liver that my doctors were watching. After being in the group for two months, I had a CAT scan that showed the spot was less defined. When I had my last CAT scan after five months in Dr. Sha's group, my doctors couldn't see the spot!"

Cancer friends can not only recover, they can actually heal others as they do so with the power of their own blocked energy that's being released. Experiments have proven that our bodies emit waves of energy, energy that can be channeled into others. "Few people are aware of the substantial but invisible energy links that exist within themselves and between others,"[2] writes Dr. Leon Hammer in *Dragon Rises, Red Bird Flies*. As a number of cancer survivors have already mentioned, directing the excess energy responsible for their cancerous cells toward someone else can prove beneficial to both parties. Indeed, because people with cancer have greater accumulations of this excess energy than others, they also have greater healing potential. In fact, cancer friends are the best healers.

HEALING SELF—AND OTHERS

This turnaround in terms of one's self-identity—from patient/victim to healer—is another important step along the road to recovery.

"I have been diagnosed with breast cancer, but I decided not to do chemotherapy. Instead, I asked the gods and goddesses to help me find a different way to heal and was told about Drs. Sha and Gray's self-healing group," writes Letty. "This has been a miracle for my healing. There was intensive energy work and a great deal of emotional support. The positive way of thinking and being was a very welcome and refreshing relief. For my healing, I have abandoned a victim mentality and know I am now working for my health. I have learned how to help heal my own cancer using the power self-healing techniques. I have learned how to help heal others. As a cancer sufferer, I have learned that the excess energy around my cancer cells can be a powerful force for self-healing and healing. It only needs to be directed properly.

"This feels absolutely right to my inner self. Putting more magic back into my everyday life is like a homecoming for me and, after a few short months, my sickness is gone! Healing and living a beautiful life is now my goal for my soul. Being in this group feels so good—a different kind of support, a *doing* (a healing) as well as good words and thoughts. Active participation in your own healing as well as helping others—how empowering!"

Many people report being able to heal loved ones despite the many miles that separate them. Remember Jerry, the colon-cancer survivor whose self-healing efforts belied his oncologist's dire predictions?

"My ninety-year-old mother-in-law began having trouble walking and progressively got worse until she was unable to get out of bed," Jerry says. "Because she was totally unable to take care of herself at this point, the family began to make arrangements

for some outside care. That night I decided to practice some distance healing. I was in California and my mother-in-law was in
Wisconsin. I crawled into bed, and in a reverent, quiet, profound
state of peace I called upon the souls of all the great healers,
Buddha, Jesus, and Mary to assist in the healing and asked for the
cell soul, organ soul, and the body soul of my mother-in-law to
help. I visualized blue, white, and gold light descending through
her body, through all her cells, organs, muscles, and nerves, energizing her whole body with a healing light. Then the lights
formed three balls of light in the body, one of gold light in the
head, one of white light in the lungs, and one blue light in the
abdomen. I remember thinking that these lights would always be
in her body to be called upon at any time to do whatever healing
her body needed to do. Any additional energy the body needed
would naturally call upon these lights whenever needed. I closed
with '*Hao! Hao! Hao!* Thank you! Thank you! Thank you!'
Thanking the great souls for coming, I then drifted off to sleep.
The next morning my wife called her brother in Wisconsin, and
he said it was like a miracle because my mother-in-law was up
walking around like the Energizer Bunny."

You already know almost all the power self-healing techniques
you need to effect these kinds of profound changes in yourself
and others. Allow me to share just one last one with you.

The One Hand Self-Healing Method is a simple, practical,
powerful, and profound technique created by the founder of Zhi
Neng medicine, Master and Dr. Zhi Chen Guo, to self-heal cancer and many other unhealthy conditions.

How does it work?

When you point the tips of your fingers at the cancerous area,
the energy from your fingers radiates to the cancer cells to make
them vibrate fast. This causes the energy accumulation between

the cancer cells to dissipate and flow to other parts of the body. The energy density in the space between the cells is reduced and dissipates. When the highly accumulated energy around cancer cells dissipates, you need not worry. The cancer cells themselves are not transferred to other parts of the body. It's the energy around the cancer cells that is transferred to nourish other parts of the body. When this energy flow continues, the cancer cells will gradually transform back into normal cells.

Healing Practice: One Hand Self-Healing Method
Prepare (Body Power Technique)

Relax in any comfortable position. You may stand, sit, or lie down.

Hand Position (Body Power Technique)

Point the fingers and thumb of one hand at the cancerous area, holding it 12 to 20 inches away. If you have more than one cancerous area, practice this exercise separately for each area.

Communicate (Soul Power Technique)

"I love the soul of [name the cancerous area]. Please help transfer the excess energy to other parts of my body."

Visualize (Mind Power Technique)

Visualize bright white light radiating in the cancerous area. Visualize the area as transparent and healthy.

Chant (Sound Power Technique)

Chant the sounds of the special healing number mantra 3396815 ("sahn sahn joe lew bah yow woo") as fast as you can, for as long as you can.

Close (Soul Power Technique)

"*Hao, hao, hao.* Thank you, thank you, thank you."

Practice Time

Practice three to five minutes each time. Cancer is a serious condition. Practice many times a day.

Though each person's cancer is waste (at best) for his or her own body, it's actually a nutrient for another person. You can use this same method to partner with someone else who has cancer simply by pointing to each other's cancerous areas, visualizing a light radiating in those spots, and rapidly chanting "Light, light, light, light" either aloud or silently. Keep this up for three minutes at a time, and then repeat as often as you can every day. As with any and all of the power self-healing techniques, you want to close each session with the statement of hope and gratitude, "*Hao, hao, hao.* Thank you, thank you, thank you."

For Jackie, whose recovery shows us how joyful self-healing can be, learning about the potential and power to heal others—and seeing that perhaps there was a profound reason behind her cancer—proved the greatest reward.

"Sometimes an illness like cancer makes you feel so serious and sad that you don't want to live. Healing begins when we remember the feeling of being healthy, but everyone still looks at you like you're sick. The tombstones of despair, the graveyards of failures that I had walked through were bleak. I did not need to feel like I was dead in my recovery period. Finding out that I possessed the power to heal others gave me a renewed sense of purpose and power and the passion to live, because each time I would quietly send healing energy to someone by visualizing light, they would improve.

"Dr. Sha's message that cancer sufferers are the best healers is really powerful and gives us a new potential identity. Creating such a profound positive out of an illness is not only restorative; it's intensely healing."

To close this chapter, I want to share one last story of hope and transformation from a cancer survivor named Willie.

"I'm a truck driver who is very close to retirement. When my wife first heard about Dr. Sha, we were both dealing with high blood pressure. We wanted a way to manage our blood pressure without medication, which always seems to have side effects. Figuring I had nothing to lose, I accompanied my wife to Dr. Sha's presentation.

"We were both very impressed with Dr. Sha's energy, compassion, and joy. The healings he did on the spot were also very impressive. We purchased a few of his audiotapes and books and began to practice his self-healing and energy development exercises at home, and even while driving to work. The techniques seemed to help us manage our blood pressures. Although I can't say we showed dramatic improvements (our blood pressures would rise again under stress or if we weren't careful with our diet), they were generally down. In addition, I do believe my normal EKGs were at least partly due to my daily practice with these power self-healing techniques.

"Later that year, however, I was faced with a new and different health concern. I had begun to have frequent urination and suspected that something was wrong. When I discovered blood in my urine one day, I knew something was wrong. I went to my doctor, who had me take various tests. My PSA blood test showed a level of 258, a very high level. He referred me to a cancer specialist right away who admitted me to the hospital for a biopsy. When I regained consciousness after the surgery, the specialist was there to tell me, 'You have cancer.'

"Shortly after my diagnosis, I learned Dr. Sha would be back in the area, so I went to see him five times in a two-week period for treatment. After the first three visits, when Dr. Sha explained to me that cancer cells are caused by an accumulation of excess energy and that cancer cells can return to normal cells if that excess energy is dissipated, I really didn't feel anything from his treatment. During my fourth visit, though, I really felt the energy surging through my body. My body began to rock and sway on its own as the energy moved. This was something I was totally unprepared for, and it was almost unbelievable to me. But it gave me even more faith and confidence in Dr. Sha's theories and in his healing methods.

"I began practicing more and more, and the energy in my body continued to physically move my body. This had become a normal occurrence, one that I expected and looked forward to. I was doing other things too, including taking herbs and receiving radiation treatment for my prostate. Although I was at times a little depressed, I tried to maintain a healthy lifestyle and outlook, going for daily walks with my wife. I had faith and peace in my belief that I was doing everything I could to recover. While I was on radiation, I never got sick or fatigued, always driving myself and walking up steep hills to get to the hospital. I always had lots of energy.

"After seven months, I was fully able to return to work. My PSA test after I returned to work showed a level of 1. My next test, which I had recently, showed a level of 1 again. When I told my doctor I wanted to travel as soon as I retired, he told me, 'Go! Your health is no obstacle.'

"I attribute my success in healing from prostate cancer to all of the things I did. I don't know if I would have healed as well if I'd left out any aspect of my healing. I do firmly believe that my recovery would not have happened without Dr. Sha's healing, as well as the self-healing practices that I learned from him.

"Dr. Sha has taught me that I have to give out the excess energy around my cancer cells, to help them return to normal cells. He also says that this energy can be a great nutrient for others. Now, I'm a very shy person. I could never speak in front of an audience or try to use Dr. Sha's methods directly with anybody who doesn't know and accept those methods. But I have started to use Dr. Sha's methods by 'long distance' on several members of my family, without even informing them that I'm doing this.

"What I use is the One Hand Healing Method. I calm myself and face the person, whether he or she is in Arkansas, Illinois, or wherever. Then I point the fingers of my right hand toward the person and visualize a golden healing ball or bright white light in the area where the person needs help.

"I first did this with my eighty-seven-year old mother, who had cataracts in her eyes and was in danger of losing her vision. Her doctor had told her that the only solution was eye surgery, but that she was too elderly and frail to undergo it. I sent my excess energy and light to her three or four times a week for about seven or eight weeks. When she returned to the doctor, he told her, 'I don't know how it happened, but your cataracts have cleared up. You don't have to see me any more for that problem, because it's no longer a problem!'

"Next I gave some distant healing to my brother-in-law, who had been diagnosed with terminal intestinal cancer and was told that he had only three weeks to a month to live. I have been trying to help him every day, using the same One Hand Healing Method, visualizing light nourishing his body, while at the same time receiving light from his intestines to nourish my body. It's been four weeks since the diagnosis, and my brother-in-law is still vigorous. His voice is strong and clear and he is able to walk without difficulty. His quality of life and, it seems, the length of his life are definitely exceeding his doctors' expectations. If what I'm doing is helping, I am very grateful for this wonderful blessing that I have learned from Dr. Sha.

"I've also just started to try to help other family members with rectal cancer, hepatitis C, high blood pressure, a transplanted kidney, and depression. It's too soon to report any results, but I am very hopeful that good things will happen for them.

"I always ask God to give me energy to help others. After all, isn't that what life is about?"

SHARING THE WEALTH

Cancer friends are not the only ones who have the power to heal, or the only ones who can reap the enormous benefits that come from helping others.

"When I learned to heal others—and myself in the process—I got to see a new role for my life unfold, which enhanced my sense of confidence and my ability to connect with others," says Gary, an entrepreneur and car buff. "Learning how to heal and helping people to see that they're okay gave me a whole new sense of empowerment and joy.

"My true test came when my son Kevin's girlfriend had a terrible automobile accident. She was taken by ambulance to the trauma unit and then to intensive care for weeks. Severe brain swelling and spinal injuries had placed her ninety-pound body in a life-threatened mode. One move in the wrong direction would render her paralyzed for life. My son immediately called me to the hospital, where I performed the soul power technique and called on the soul world and the soul of her organs and body to get well. Then I did the mind power technique, visualizing light in her body and seeing her as healed, perfect, and complete. I used the sound power technique and talked to her brain and the cells of her body. I told her brain to get well and her spinal cord to heal.

"Now, I can't say this made all the difference in her recovery. She had great medical care. But I will say she remembered my visits to her bedside at the hospital vividly and profoundly. The doctors released her very quickly and her rehabilitation went very fast. The family was terrified that she was going to be an invalid but, soon after, she was walking and running around again."

As we've seen time and time again, healing those around you is one of the best ways to heal yourself. "I always try to get people over the age of forty to realize that one of the greatest gifts they can give to themselves is taking time to heal other people instead of focusing on their own sicknesses," says my friend and colleague John Gray. "It's the best way there is to stay young, vibrant, and healthy, for when the energy flows through you to the person you're working with, you get the benefit as well."

There is an important spiritual law and principle in the universe: The only way to receive new knowledge and wisdom is to share the old knowledge and wisdom. It's like storing goods in a warehouse. If the warehouse is full, you can't put anything more inside. So to go on expanding your own self-healing abilities, you must share them with someone else.

Trust me, you have the power.

"I had a friend who needed ear surgery," recalls Marie, the nurse who self-healed the pulled muscle in her chest. "She had lots of liquid in her ear canal. So I did a healing for her. For twenty minutes, I chanted 'God's light,' asking the mantra to heal my friend's ear. I also visualized God's light vibrating and radiating in her ear.

"The next morning, she went to her doctor for the surgery. He looked at her and exclaimed, 'You don't need surgery! What did you do?'

"'Marie did a healing on me,'" she responded.

"'Who is Marie?' he asked. 'I want to talk to her. It's not possible! The water cannot go away like that!'

"The surgeon had twenty years of experience and had never seen a case like this. But my friend didn't have to have the surgery, which pleased and excited her to no end."

CONCLUSION

We are coming to the end of *Power Healing: The Four Keys to Energizing Your Body, Mind, and Spirit.* In conclusion, I want to offer a few points to those who want to do self-healing and take responsibility for their own well-being.

My life's journey has led me to the four keys to power healing. All of my studies have helped me understand the four keys deeply. Many of these techniques were kept secret for thousands of years in China. In ancient times, the commitment of energy and spiritual masters to their healing and spiritual journeys was lifelong. When blessed by Heaven Teams, these masters continued to discover more secret techniques. The masters would share their secrets with only a few disciples, sometimes only one. Often, the secrets were passed on only when the master was dying. Many secrets have been lost because masters did not pass them on before they died.

It took me nearly forty years of seeking, learning, and practicing to acquire the knowledge and wisdom presented to you in this book. I have had the honor and privilege of studying with great masters and teachers in many Chinese arts, from whom I received the deepest secrets and wisdom. Today, as a master myself, I am confident that this is the time to share these powerful ancient Chinese secrets and wisdom with the West and the entire world, and I am honored to do so. As you learn, practice, benefit from, and master these techniques, they—and their power—will not be secrets to you.

To learn these deep and profound techniques, held secret for so long, is a great blessing from the spiritual world. Their combination—the knowledge of how to use the four keys to power healing together—is my gift to the entire world. This has been a great blessing for the enlightenment of my own spiritual journey. I hope it will be a great blessing for yours.

I have introduced in this book only what I consider to be the most vital knowledge, wisdom, and techniques for self-healing body, mind, and soul. I selected only the most powerful body, sound, mind, and soul power techniques to offer to you, and I tried to use the simplest language to explain them. These techniques, and the concepts and theories supporting them, are simple, practical, powerful, and profound.

I believe a big change in the energy, spirit, and consciousness of the universe is coming in the twenty-first century. Knowledge and wisdom cannot be held in secret anymore. They should—and must—be opened to everybody, to benefit the entire world.

Parts of the four keys to power healing have been practiced by millions of people throughout the history of China. Through them, these people have found the "healer within." The four keys, proven effective for healing body, mind, and soul, I now offer to you, your family, and your friends. Take them. Try them. Enjoy them. Take responsibility for your own well-being by applying these techniques and practices in your daily life. Get the benefits for your health and a blessing for your life.

The power-healing techniques are offered as help for doctors and healers. These self-healing methods will help the clients of doctors, healers, psychologists, and all other health-care providers to restore their own health faster. The four keys to power healing support all other healing services. These self-healing tools will help everyone treat unhealthy conditions at the physical, emotional, and spiritual levels.

If you are in relatively good health, the techniques in this book will help you strengthen your immune system to prevent unhealthy conditions, increase your energy, improve the quality of your life, and prolong your life. If your unhealthy condition is at an early stage, power healing will help you recover relatively quickly. If you suffer chronic or life-threatening conditions, using power-healing techniques will help you restore your health much faster than using other healing methods alone.

An important spiritual law in the universe says: The only way to receive new secrets and wisdom is to share the old secrets and wisdom. It is like storing goods in a warehouse. If the warehouse is full, you can't put anything more inside. If you keep the secrets locked up and do not share them, new secrets and new knowledge cannot come in. If you share the secrets you have learned with the world, then new secrets and new knowledge will pour into your head again. Following this important spiritual law is the secret to increasing knowledge and wisdom.

If you follow the old ways and try to keep knowledge secret, you will fall behind as a teacher. If as a teacher you keep the secrets, your students will not be satisfied, and you will receive no new secrets or new knowledge. Whatever secrets you learn from this book, be generous and share them. New knowledge and new secrets will then come to you. More blessings will come to you. There are countless secrets in the universe. Sharing the old secrets to get new ones is a perfect way to acquire more wisdom, blessings, and enlightenment.

Requesting your own soul to heal your body, mind, and soul is a vital secret. Use it. Practice it sincerely and respectfully. Remember, no matter how much you learn from this book, if you want to continue acquiring new knowledge, share these techniques with your family, friends, and colleagues. Teach them how to apply the four keys to power healing together to heal themselves and bless their lives. Use the knowledge and techniques to heal and benefit each other.

Sharing knowledge and wisdom is a great virtue. Virtue is a record of service. Virtue is called *te* (pronounced "duh") in Taoist practice and karma in Buddhist practice. Accumulating virtue, *te,* or karma is one of the most important purposes of a person's life—it's the number-one issue, in fact. After you die, your soul goes to the spiritual world. Your soul does not carry any material things, such as money or property, only virtue, *te,* or karma. If you believe in reincarnation, as I do, then good virtue, *te,* or karma will bring good fortune, good health, happiness, joy, satisfaction, and success in your next life. Even if you don't believe in reincarnation, good virtue, *te,* or karma will lead your soul to a higher level of heaven.

Christians believe that God creates everything in the universe. Buddhists believe it's "emptiness," and Taoists believe it's Xu Wu, meaning "nothingness." Confucians say it's heaven, and the majority of ordinary people in China believe it's Lao Tian Ye, or "Old Heaven Grandfather." Muslims credit Allah, and Hindus think it's Shiva who creates everything in the universe.

Although each belief system has its own name for God, I personally believe that there is only one God. I am speaking frankly here and merely sharing a personal belief. If you agree with me, that's fine. If you disagree with me, please forgive me and keep your own belief system. We have no time to argue with one another. Whether you are religious or not, power healing will work for you. Let us respect each other. Let us love each other. Let us join hands together to create a new world.

There is a very powerful statement in Chinese energy, spiritual, and martial arts study: *Shi fu ling jin men; xiu xing zai ge ren.* Translation: "The master brings you in the door. How deep you go, how successful you are, how powerful you are in your life and spiritual journey depends on you." This book will bring you and many others in the self-healing door. How successful you are, once inside, depends on you.

The spiritual world contains unlimited knowledge and wisdom. One of the best ways to gain access to it is to open your spiritual communication channels, such as the Message Center, to converse with your Heaven Team. Another way is to open your Third Eye to see your Heaven Team and to receive the knowledge they can pass on to you.

Learn from your teachers how to open your Message Center and Third Eye; let your teachers bring you in the door. After you have acquired the ability to communicate directly with your Heaven Team and God, you can receive knowledge directly from them. Learning directly from your Heaven Team and God is vital for making progress on your spiritual journey.

If you have studied the concepts and practiced the techniques presented in this book, you know how to use the four keys to power healing together to build up your foundation energy centers, promote and balance your energy flow, and heal your body, mind, and soul. This book can bring you in the door of your healing and spiritual journey. Open your spiritual communication channels and learn directly from countless spiritual teachers in the universe. If you do, your journey will be blessed and enlightened, your understanding of spiritual principles and laws will continue to grow, and every moment in your life will be filled with peace, joy, and satisfaction.

Self-healing will be one of the major health issues in the twenty-first century. At the beginning of this new century, this book offers you practical tools to self-heal. The techniques you have learned have served millions of people in China throughout history. I believe they are going to serve millions of people in the West and in the entire world in the years to come. The four keys to power healing are the means of nourishing your health. The universe blesses these tools, this nourishment, to the benefit of all human beings in the entire world. By applying body power, sound power, mind power, and soul power techniques together, as I have shown you, you will begin to experience the greatest benefits. Some of you will see significant changes in body, mind, and soul right away. Recovery from chronic illness, chronic pain, and life-threatening diseases takes more time. Continue your healing activities with your health-care professionals, but be sure to practice self-healing techniques as well.

The four keys to power healing are in your hands now. Study them. Digest them. Practice them to benefit your health; to heal your body, mind, and soul; to bless your relationships and your success; and to enlighten your spiritual journey. I wish you great health, happiness, enjoyment, and success in your life.

Let everybody in the entire world join hands to create a healthy, happy, peaceful, satisfied, and enlightened twenty-first century. Bless your health and bless your journey.

Thank you. Thank you. Thank you.

God's blessing.

Your Heaven Team's blessing.

Your soul's blessing.

ACKNOWLEDGMENTS

In April 2000, I was invited to speak at the Whole Life Expo in San Francisco. A man came to my display and asked, "Is this the booth for Dr. Sha?" Although I had no idea who he was, my assistants recognized him and told me he was a very well-known and highly-respected author. He continued, "I would like to attend your presentation tomorrow."

I responded, "You are welcome to join us."

As I would learn shortly afterward from my assistants, this is how I met John Gray, relationship expert and author of *Men Are from Mars, Women Are from Venus* and many other best-selling books.

The next day, I gave my presentation in which I demonstrated the power-healing techniques in this book. The techniques gave relief on the spot to attendees with shoulder pain and back pain. Then John Gray volunteered to receive power healing for his chronic foot pain. He was amazed by the results.

Later that day, I in turn attended John's presentation at the Expo and felt incredible energy from his speaking and healing. This is how we started to become acquainted. He asked me, "Have you written any books?"

I replied, "Yes, I've written a few self-published books."

John further urged me, "Dr. Sha, you have great healing capabilities and wonderful healing wisdom. Why don't you write a new book about healing?"

The following month, I returned to San Francisco to teach. John attended my workshops, and we got to know each other better. He told me, "If I can help you in any way with your new book, I will." From the start, John gave me great encouragement and support. I am now honored to call him a good friend. I am deeply grateful for his contribution of the Foreword to this book. From the bottom of my heart, I deeply acknowledge and thank him for all of his great efforts and support on my behalf. Without John's efforts, HarperCollins would not have published this book.

I'm very blessed and honored to have an excellent and most supportive editor at HarperSanFrancisco, Gideon Weil. He has done so much for me through the whole process of creating this book. We have had many productive meetings and telephone conversations. I have always felt his great care for my book. He has consistently demonstrated his fine editorial capabilities. He has always communicated openly with my team and me and he has listened with an open and receptive mind to our suggestions. From my heart, I thank him for all his support, which I know comes from his heart. I am grateful that God sent me such an excellent editor.

Gideon introduced me to Linden Gross, an editor, writer, and journalist who has ghostwritten a recent best-seller and several other significant books. A successful author herself, Linden made a huge contribution by suggesting that I add many more personal stories of how people have benefited from power healing. She has also done an excellent job with the overall structure and organization of my book, as well as with the personal stories and the research on complementary and alternative medicine. I value her contributions greatly.

I deeply appreciate Stephen Hanselman, publisher, Margery Buchanan, marketing director, Kathi Goldmark, senior marketing and publicity manager, Eric Brandt, associate director of marketing and publicity, and Chris Hafner, production editor at HarperSanFrancisco, as well as Diane Reverand, senior vice president at HarperCollins, all of whom were most supportive and helpful.

Jacqueline Miller was responsible for most of the background research, and also did an excellent job collecting, editing, and working closely with Linden on many of the personal stories. Jackie, with her husband Andrew Michael, supported me closely for a few months in many other areas of my beginning journey in the United States, and is continuing to help in some critical areas. From my heart, I appreciate all of her efforts on my behalf.

Two special people invited me as a guest in their homes so that I could work on the book in a peaceful, pleasant, and private environment. Mari Bittick let me stay in her home for about two months. She not only gave me a room to stay and work in, she also very generously cared for me. I thank her deeply for her unconditional support.

I would also like to show particular appreciation and gratitude to Anita Meier, who gave me the use of one of her homes for ten months. For such great support and generosity, despite her own major health issues, I cannot thank her enough.

I'm also very blessed and honored to have had some dedicated students help me with this book. Without them, this book would not be in your hands.

Two of these students, Ida Berk and Peggy Werner, have studied with me for a few years. When I began to write this book, Ida saw immediately that I needed help. Although I can converse comfortably in English, I need help with grammar, spelling and vocabulary in my writing. Ida left her job and assisted me day and night for months. For her great dedication, I cannot thank her enough.

Peggy also helped me day and night for months. In addition to editing the book, she assisted me in many other ways for a few years. She shared her home for my teaching, handled communications with my clients and students, and organized events for me. For all of her efforts, I cannot thank her enough.

I would like to give a very special appreciation and acknowledgement to Allan Chuck. He came to me in April 2000 with his wife Mimi. Together, they attended a few of my workshops, then began to help Ida, Peggy, and me on my book. I immediately saw that Allan had great editing capabilities. I also saw that Mimi always had great ideas to contribute as well. Without Ida, Peggy, and Allan, this book would not be available to serve you. My deepest appreciation goes to them.

Allan became dedicated to helping on my book and other things, devoting many hours every day. Shortly thereafter, and until recently, as my organization grew significantly, Allan became the main person to handle almost all of my activities. He has been fully dedicated to supporting all aspects of my life for almost two years now, without asking for or expecting anything from me. He is the most dedicated assistant and devoted student I have, and he is a true friend. I would also like to express my deep appreciation for Mimi. Her integrity and devotion to support me are deeply moving. Without her dedicated support, Allan would not have been able to make such a huge contribution to my life. For their total dedication and support, I will appreciate Mimi and Allan for a lifetime.

I would also like to give deep appreciation from my heart to several other wonderful people.

Anita Meier also introduced me to her close friends Harry Youtt and Judith Prager, both great writers and teachers. They came from Los Angeles to San Francisco specifically to volunteer their support and offered many constructive editorial suggestions to Ida, Peggy, Allan, and me. For their many hours of great support, I give them special acknowledgment and deep thanks. I cannot thank them enough.

In the final phases of editing, my dear friend Dr. Po Chi Wu gave me many critical and valuable suggestions. I appreciate him and his contributions very highly. I would also like to acknowledge his lovely wife, Mary Thé, for giving me a place in her beautiful office to do private consultations for more than a year. Mary has also introduced me to many clients, several of whom are now giving me great support as well. Anytime I need Po Chi and Mary's help on any issue, they are there for me right away. They support me unconditionally from their hearts. I feel in my heart that they are my dear brother and sister. I cannot thank Po Chi and Mary enough.

Marie Lehrer has helped with so many things during the last year-and-a-half. Her unconditional devotion to serve people and her energetic support of my work really touch me. She has made possible many opportunities for me to teach at hospitals, universities, and bookstores. She always offers sincere suggestions and good ideas. I can't thank her enough.

Sabita Suedat and Robert Lewis gave me great support in Toronto with dictation, typing, and editing of some of my teachings. As dedicated students, they have also supported me in many other ways. I deeply appreciate them both.

Other very important supporters in Canada include May Guey Chew, Diana Holland, Steven James Wong, Sharon Soubolsky, Brigida Milne, and Raymond Jefferd. They were instrumental in editing and producing my first four English-language books, which were self-published.

May was the key editor and writer on these four books *(Zhi Neng Medicine: Revolutionary Self-Healing Methods from China,* which is in many ways a predecessor to this book, *Soul Study: A Guide to Accessing Your Highest Powers, Sha's Golden Healing Ball: The Perfect Gift,* and *Numbers 0 to 108: Messages to Enhance Your Life).* She devoted a few years of her life to support me unconditionally. She also gathered personal stories for this book from many of my Canadian students. For her dedication and most valuable contributions to my books and work, I thank her for a lifetime.

Diana Holland is an excellent editor. She provided incredible editorial input for my earlier books. Diana, May, and Steven, whom I also deeply appreciate, collaborated on the final editing. Sharon and Brigida used their communication channels to the spiritual world to give me great assistance in writing *Numbers 0 to 108.* Raymond contributed to the final editing of *Sha's Golden Healing Ball.* To all of them, I give my deeply heartfelt thanks.

I would like to thank a few other Canadian students for their great support of my work: Dr. Yuan Yuan, Cicily Fowlie, Giok Khoen Khoe, Thai-Siew Liang, Tammy Tran, and Fu Wei. There are many others not listed here, to whom I am also deeply grateful.

In my brief time in San Francisco, I have had a dedicated group of medical doctors and students who have given great support to the cancer research group created and headed by John Gray and me.

As the medical director for our research, Dr. Than Aw, supported by Ida Berk, helped design the Cancer Recovery Pilot Study. Our research team also included Dr. Blesilda Liganor, Dr. Elizabeth Targ, and Dr. Peter Hudoba. Dr. Hudoba contributed a great deal of effort to analyze, document, and present, with Ida, the study results at the First World Symposium on Self-Healing last year. The entire team gave great input to all aspects of the study. Gary Elliott and Rebecca Dugan were totally dedicated every week to our research sessions, even leading the power healing for extended periods when I could not be present in person. I am most appreciative of Jackie Miller's efforts in helping me obtain space at the Presidio Alliance Community Center, and offer great thanks to Leanne Hoadley, Executive Director and Jessy Buttrick, Events Coordinator of the Presidio Alliance, for very kindly donating their facility to our research at no cost for several months.

More recently, Dr. Wyndolyn Barnes has joined our cancer research team and assumed many responsibilities. Others who have been dedicated to the research efforts include Dr. Aubrey Degnan, Shu Chin Hsu, Marie Lehrer, Rita Chang, Tom and Donna Vickers, Dr. Janedare Winston, Jennifer Tayloe, Addy Murphy, Dr. Theresa Steinberg, and Anita Eubank. I thank them all for their great support.

To all of the participants in the research studies, I extend my heartfelt compassion for your health issues and my deep appreciation for your faith in and support of Zhi Neng medicine and power healing.

Elisa Celli has put her heart into supporting my work. She has worked closely with HarperCollins to develop and implement effective promotion and marketing plans for this book. She has introduced me to many valuable people in my journey. I deeply appreciate her efforts.

One of the special people Elisa introduced me to is George Mateljan, to whom I would like to express my deepest appreciation. George invited Elisa and me to stay in his home in Hawaii and treated me like a son. His unconditional love and support of my power-healing journey touch me deeply. I will forever be grateful for his love and care.

George in turn introduced me to Christina Fisher and Jerome Kellner, who organized very successful power healing and teaching events for me in Maui. They did an excellent job, for which I thank them very much.

I also greatly appreciate Francisco Gomes, who shared his deep spiritual gifts with me while I was in Maui. I hold the gift of his sharing in the greatest esteem. I cannot thank him enough.

In my current power healing work, I would like to extend special appreciation to many other dedicated supporters, including Sam Chang, Evi Kahle, Tom McConnell, Mark "Doc" Lane, and Sarah Alexander.

I would like to express my deepest appreciation to Elizabeth Enright. For the last few years, she has helped me greatly with editorial support, for this book and for *Numbers 0 to 108.* She is an excellent editor. I deeply appreciate and value her great contribution.

As the attorney for my organization, Jack Russo has been most generous with his support. His legal and business insights are always penetrating and most valuable. His lovely wife Carol also supports us from her heart. I value both of them greatly.

Dr. Faudry Pierre-Louis wrote the foreword to *Zhi Neng Medicine.* He and his wife, Carmen, have given me very valuable support for my power healing work in Canada. I am deeply grateful for both of them.

I would especially like to honor Dr. Donald W. Stewart and his late wife Marnie. He is a pioneer of alternative medicine and preventive medicine in Canada. He has supported my work unconditionally in many ways and helped me with scientific research on chronic pain. I cannot thank him enough.

Francesco Garripoli, who filmed me and my master and teacher, Dr. Zhi Chen Guo, for his PBS documentary, *Qigong— Ancient Chinese Healing for the 21st Century,* has introduced me to many influential people and organizations in the world of qigong. He and his wife, Daisy, have given me great support from the bottom of their hearts for the last few years, especially his work for this book and for creating my Web site, www.drsha.com. They are like brother and sister to me. I cannot thank them enough.

I deeply appreciate Barbara Bernie, who has given me such great support for many aspects of my work. She is a person of the highest integrity and great sincerity. I am honored to have her and her husband Norman as such great friends.

Sylvia Chen, her husband, Dr. Wen-Hsiung Chen, and their lovely children, Alan and Angela, have supported me since they met me in 1992. Sylvia has organized many of my trips to the United States, Taiwan, China, Vancouver, Montreal, and many other cities to spread my teaching of Zhi Neng medicine and power healing. She is the one who has given me the greatest contribution to my journey. Even though her family is in Canada, I know their hearts are with me. Sylvia has already visited me three times during my brief time in San Francisco to give me her direct support and guidance. Dr. Chen is a professor of physics who wrote the "To the Reader" section in *Zhi Neng Medicine.* He shared his great scientific knowledge with me in reviewing the theoretical concepts in this book. For their unconditional wholehearted support of my journey, I will thank Sylvia and her family for my lifetime.

Laurie Macabasco generously shared her artistic talents for the illustrations in this book. I give Laurie my warmest thanks for her kind support.

Lois Tema provided the photographs for this book. For her professionalism and dedication to quality, I am most appreciative.

To the many people who have generously shared personal stories of their experiences with power healing, I express my deep appreciation. This includes those whose stories appear in this book, as well as those whose stories are not included here. Thank you for your openness to power healing and for your willingness to inspire hope in others by sharing your successes.

To the many others who have supported me in any aspect of this book or my work, whom I may have inadvertently forgotten to mention, although I do not list you by name, I deeply appreciate and value all your contributions.

If there is knowledge and wisdom in this book that will serve you, I must acknowledge all the great masters and teachers from whom I have learned so much. I thank my Chinese philosophy teacher in Toronto, Professor Qiu Yun Lee, my Buddhist master in Taiwan, Wu Yi, and my I Ching and feng shui master, Professor Da Jun Liu at Shandong University in China, for all their great education and guidance. My special appreciation and highest respect go to Master and Dr. Zhi Chen Guo, my teacher and adoptive father, from whom I have learned the most, and to his wife Jin Jie Jiang and their five daughters. Dr. Guo's teaching, knowledge, and wisdom form the foundation for this book.

Finally, I acknowledge my loving family. To my wife, Dr. Qion Xi Luo, our sweet and lovely children Sherina, Stephanie, and Anthony, my father, Bai Lu Sha, my mother, Yi Chuan Zhang, my father-in-law, Jing Ting Luo, and my mother-in-law, Zhi He Cao, my brother and sisters, and their families, my wife's brothers and sister and their families, I thank you so much for your unconditional love and support without which I could not accomplish my life's mission.

NOTES

CHAPTER 2
1. Leon Hammer, *Dragon Rises, Red Bird Flies* (Talman, 1991), p. 3.
2. Ibid., p. 5.

CHAPTER 6
1. Herbert Benson, *The Relaxation Response* (Avon, 1990), p. xi.
2. Benson, *Relaxation Response,* p. 59.

CHAPTER 7
1. Relax the anus after the initial squeeze. Make no effort to focus on this through-out the practice. The purpose of contracting the anus initially is to connect the four meridians (*du, ren, chong,* and *dai*) that cross paths in the Snow Mountain Area, a key energy center of the body. This allows the energy that develops through this body power technique to flow through all four meridians.

CHAPTER 8
1. The Mandarin Chinese pronunciation of the number and healing sounds used in Zhi Neng medicine works best for healing and energy development, as described. But because the message is associated with the meanings as well as the sounds, saying them in another language still sends healing messages to stimulate the organs.

CHAPTER 9
1. Joan Borysenko, *Minding the Body, Mending the Mind* (Bantam, 1987), p. 209.
2. Herbert Benson, *The Relaxation Response* (Avon, 1990), p. xxviii.
3. Ibid.
4. Dennis and Joyce Lawson, *Five Elements of Acupuncture and Chinese Massage* (Northamptonshire, Great Britain: Health Science Press, 1973), p. 90.

CHAPTER 10
1. Donna Eden and David Feinstein, *Energy Medicine* (Tarcher/Putnam, 1998), p. 20.

CHAPTER 13
1. Andrew Weil, *Spontaneous Healing* (Ballantine, 1995), p. 252.
2. American Medical Association, *Essential Guide to Depression* (Pocket Books, 1998), p. 14 and Sung Son and Jeffrey Kirchner, *Depression in Children and Adolescents* (American Family Physician, Vol. 62, No. 10).
3. Roger Jahnke, *The Healer Within* (HarperSanFrancisco, 1997), pp. 176–78.

CHAPTER 14
1. Andrew Weil, *Spontaneous Healing* (Ballantine, 1995), p. 129.
2. Leon Hammer, *Dragon Rises, Red Bird Flies* (Talman, 1991), p. 87.